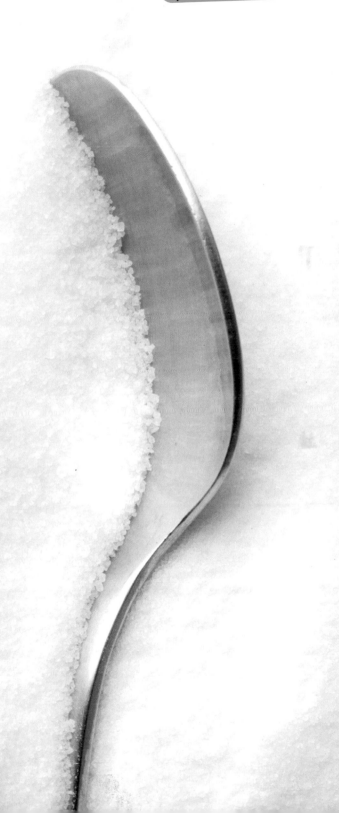

First published in 2013 by Victory Belt Publishing Inc.

ISBN-13: 978-1-936608-13-3

The information included in this book is for educational purposes only. It is not intended or implied to be a substitute for professional medical advice. The reader should always consult his or her healthcare provider to determine the appropriateness of the information for his or her own situation or with any questions regarding a medical condition or treatment plan. Reading the information in this book does not create a physician-patient relationship.

Book design: Joan Olkowski, Graphic D-signs, Inc.
Food photography: Diane Sanfilippo & Tonja Field
Cover portrait: Kelli Beavers
Hair: Samantha Gaiser
Make-up: Hayley Mason

Printed in Canada
TC 0819

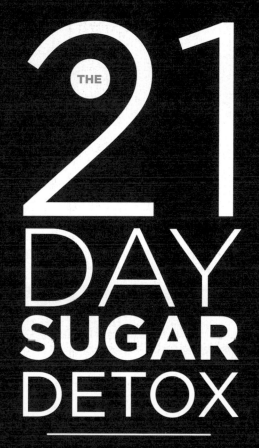

THE 21 DAY SUGAR DETOX

OVER 100 RECIPES
FOR ANY PROGRAM LEVEL

COOKBOOK

DIANE SANFILIPPO, BS, NC

VICTORY BELT PUBLISHING INC.
LAS VEGAS

TABLE OF CONTENTS

The 21-Day Sugar Detox Cookbook

SECTION 1

introduction

The 21-Day Sugar Detox

"Things do not change; we change." —Henry David Thoreau

About me

Hi there. I'm Diane Sanfilippo. I'm a certified holistic nutrition consultant. And, like you, I've struggled with sugar and carb cravings. Sugar is such a powerful force that I too had trouble breaking through to the other side—to sugar *freedom*. But I have found the solution to this huge problem, and I've never felt better!

I created The 21-Day Sugar Detox program because curbing sugar and carb cravings has become a top priority for those seeking a healthier path in life. In my practice over the years, I've worked with countless clients, both one-on-one and in large groups, who've struggled with sugar and carb cravings. In fact, I created my practice with blood sugar regulation as a primary focus in order to help people just like you.

The 21-Day Sugar Detox is great for anyone who wants to take control of sugar cravings—from busy moms to competitive athletes. It's for anyone who wants to feel better, increase energy, improve sleep, and break the cycle of being on a blood sugar roller coaster (you know, the ride you're on when your meals and snacks are rich in carbs and lacking in vitamins and minerals) all day long.

In a world where conflicting diet advice comes at us from every angle—from television doctors, magazines, the evening news, and even your hairdresser!—it's no wonder you still haven't figured out how to get your cravings under control. What you don't need is another book to tell you why sugar is harmful—you've probably read all those already, but they don't outline a clear path away from the problem. The 21-Day Sugar Detox gives you exactly that: a simple, straightforward, and practical plan to break free from the chains that sugar and carbs have wrapped tightly around you.

About The 21-Day Sugar Detox

The 21DSD is a whole-foods-based program created to help you reset your habits, your taste buds, and your *entire relationship* with the food that's on your plate every single day. After three weeks of eating the foods on The 21DSD "Yes" list, you won't be able to look at the foods you previously ate the same way. Your habits will change, along with your awareness of how certain foods make you feel. (Hint: Sweets usually leave you tired, moody, and just plain off-kilter.)

A day or two into most nutritional reset or detox programs, many people struggle with motivation—and rightly so! Most programs out there have you cutting calories, popping pills, or chugging shakes or juices all day long to achieve the desired result. But that's not *at all* what *The 21-Day Sugar Detox* is about. That type of deprivation is not what your body needs when you're looking for a fresh start—it needs clean, healthy,

Why eliminate sugar from your diet?

Sugar is a sneaky thing. It doesn't just cause cravings and make you fat; consuming too much of it can lead to all kinds of health issues, both in the short term and in the long term. Most of us are well aware of some of the common signs of sugar addiction and its deleterious effects on our lives, from extreme energy highs and lows to that nagging feeling that you won't be satisfied until you eat something sweet. But sugar's harmful effects are even more far-reaching. Here are a handful of less-obvious signs of sugar addiction, chronically erratic blood sugar levels, and nutrient deficiencies that may be caused by overconsumption of nutrient-poor carbohydrate foods:

SHORT-TERM EFFECTS
- Mood swings
- Acne, rashes
- Premenstrual syndrome (PMS), painful periods
- Unrestful sleep
- Fatigue
- Muscle fatigue or weakness
- Susceptibility to colds and flu
- Other food addictions

LONG-TERM EFFECTS
- Anemia
- Depression, anxiety
- Cystic acne, eczema, psoriasis
- PCOS, infertility
- Insomnia
- Adrenal fatigue or dysfunction
- Vision impairment
- Neurological disorders
- Insulin resistance, type 2 diabetes
- Alzheimer's disease
- Substance abuse

Whether we realize it or not, sugar is taking over our lives. From cravings and impulsive eating to the highs and lows of riding the blood sugar roller coaster, we've nearly become slaves to sweet and carb-rich foods. Now, it's not that *all* carbs are bad—quite the contrary. There are some amazing carbohydrate-rich foods out there, like vegetables and fruits, but we all know that those aren't the types of foods that cause us to spiral out of control and run for the nearest candy bowl. That's because they're what I call "good carbs." They carry calories from carbohydrates as well as vitamins and minerals that your body needs to feel satisfied and calm. There's a lot more to the good-carbs-versus-bad-carbs story than I'm explaining here, so I recommend that you reread the first portion of *The 21-Day Sugar Detox* guidebook to brush up on that information.

whole foods that are rich in nutrients. Adequate protein and fat, along with a density of vitamins and minerals in every bite, set up your body's natural detoxification system for success. You see, your body was built with the innate ability to detoxify itself! It's almost like magic, but it's really just basic biology. In order to carry out that detox process, though, you need to feed your body real food. Period.

About this cookbook

This cookbook serves as a companion and a complement to *The 21-Day Sugar Detox* guidebook, my first publication in this series. After many years of successfully running the program without printed materials for participants, I decided that it was time to make this information available in a much bigger, better way. So I wrote *The 21-Day Sugar Detox* to put all my best sugar-busting advice in one place.

The guidebook includes:

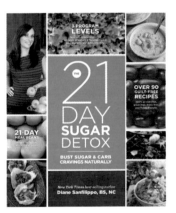

- the background science on why we crave sugar and what it does to our bodies

- how to prepare

- a day-by-day accounting of what to expect

- helpful hints and tricks for replacing foods and dining out

- where to find help and support along the way

- more than 90 easy and delicious recipes

Yes, the guidebook itself contains a *ton* of recipes. But if I've learned *anything* in the last several years about how to best support those on The 21DSD, it's that preparation and inspirational recipes are the keys to your success!

In this cookbook, you'll find over 100 more satisfying and deliciously sugar-free recipes that also gluten-free, grain-free, dairy-free, and Paleo-friendly. After completing the recipes for the first book, I realized that there are many more foods that you'll want to eat while on the program, but finding them in 21DSD-friendly recipes, well, that isn't always easy. In this book's recipes, you'll find more creative ways to enjoy your 21DSD-friendly fruits, more smoothie ideas, more egg-free breakfasts (for those who are allergic or sensitive to eggs), more flavorful main dishes, and more sides, snacks, and not-sweet treats to tempt your palate. I've also created more sugar-detox-friendly versions of your favorite dressings and sauces, along with spice blends to keep everything on your plate bursting with flavor (without the added sugars and chemical preservatives found in most commercial varieties), whether you decide to follow a specific recipe or not. The spice blends are your secret weapon and your express train to Flavor Town!

One of the best things you'll experience while on The 21-Day Sugar Detox is a remarkable change in the way your palate responds to food. After a few days, foods that did not seem that sweet before will suddenly be much sweeter. A not-sweet treat that you may have created on Day 1 will taste far more delicious by Day 7. Your taste buds will *change*—and I show you how to use that shift to your advantage in this book. Many of these recipes make use of items like caramelized onions and cooked-down green apples in sauces and dishes that you might normally sweeten with a concentrated sweetener like honey or maple syrup (which you aren't going to use while on The 21DSD). I'm talking about BBQ Sauce, a No-Honey Mustard, and even a Sweetener-Free Ketchup. You won't miss all those added sweeteners you've given up for one moment!

About the meal plans

The 21-Day Sugar Detox guidebook includes three 21-day meal plans for you to follow if you choose, based on the recipes in the book. This cookbook follows that same approach, but using only recipes from this book. These meal plans provide alternatives and expanded ideas and resources for completing your 21DSD. Whether you're tackling the detox for the first time and you simply want as many recipes at your fingertips as possible, or you're coming back for another round of The 21DSD months after completing it for the first time, I've got you covered.

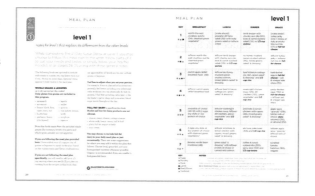

Now, you may be wondering why someone would want or need to complete The 21DSD more than once. You may think that the purpose is to rid yourself of cravings once and for all, end of story. Well, for many people, that is exactly what happens! Those three weeks can be miraculous and life-changing. Some decide to come back to The 21DSD simply to support a friend or loved one in their detox journey. But for others, especially those who enter the program at Level 1, attempting a nutritional reset a couple of times each year (and possibly at a higher level) brings on a new set of challenges and new results.

I invite you to revisit The 21DSD whenever you feel like you've gotten off-track or somehow lost sight of your sugar intake. Though you'll likely curb the vast majority of your sugar cravings in just three weeks on the program, if you decide to indulge over the holidays, for example, you may find that a post-holiday 21DSD is exactly what you need to set yourself straight again.

About the recipes

The recipes in this book are divided into the following sections:

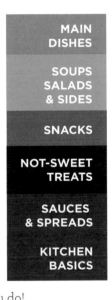

- Main Dishes

- Soups, Salads, & Sides

- Snacks

- Not-Sweet Treats

- Sauces & Spreads

- Kitchen Basics

In each section, you'll find a variety of recipes that cater to a broad spectrum of tastes and preferences. You don't need to make every recipe in this book to be successful on your detox, but you'll have a tasty time cooking your way through them if you do!

The Main Dishes section is organized with egg-free breakfasts first, then breakfast items that contain eggs. Following are poultry, red meat, pork, and seafood/meat-free options. Many of the main dishes were created along with sides that are listed in the following section, but you are welcome to mix and match them to your own tastes and preferences.

Soups, salads, and sides come next, with a variety of each and flavor profiles to suit a range of palates. Feel free to create your own easy vegetable sides or to mix and match the recipes in this book with your own go-to favorites.

Snacks are a hot topic with those who undertake The 21DSD, so I've created a new set of make-ahead savory recipes that'll keep you stocked up and prepared for when unexpected hunger hits.

Not-sweet treats are a signature (and fan favorite) of The 21-Day Sugar Detox program. Giving up old favorites for three weeks can seem overwhelming, but these re-creations will have you jumping for joy. Some of them are not going to taste as amazing on Day 1 as they will later in your detox (as I mentioned earlier, your tastes *will* change—and I'm counting on that for you!), but all of them are filled with ingredients that will nourish your body while comforting your soul.

The Kitchen Basics section includes foundational recipes upon which you'll build other recipes throughout the book. This section includes broths, sauces, spice blends, and dairy-free milk recipes that will have you wondering why you ever bought the canned, bottled, boxed, and prepackaged versions!

Using the recipes

Each recipe in this book (as well as in the guidebook) is suited for all three levels of the program and has several parts to it. You'll find the expected information, like how long it takes to make the recipe, along with the ingredient list, preparation method, and how many servings it yields. You'll also find helpful tips and tricks about ingredients, cooking techniques, and even some special equipment you'll need. Since I know how important it is for many of you to avoid certain categories of commonly allergenic or irritating foods, I've called out when a recipe contains nuts, eggs, nightshades, FODMAPs, or seafood (see pages 224-225 for more information). I've even given you notes on what to omit from the recipe if you're avoiding those foods, if the recipe will work without them. Check out the boxes for specific tips that pertain to each recipe, or turn to pages 224-225 for a complete list of ingredient swaps to use when avoiding common allergens.

You'll likely find some ingredients that are unfamiliar to you, unless you've already cooked your way through the guidebook (or my first book, *Practical Paleo*). I've created a list of special ingredients on pages 14–15 so that you can learn more about these items—what they are, why to use them, and how much to eat while on the program. A handy guide to recommended products and brands is featured on pages 226–227 so that you can discover new brands and track down unique items for your new way of eating—during the detox and beyond!

Recipe elements and how to use them

1 Recipe category indicates the type of dish it is. Note that some main dishes also include sides.

2 Recipe name, prep and cook time, servings, and yield where applicable. Servings are especially important when considering allowed portions of included fruits.

3 Allergens included in the recipe as-written. If an ingredient is optional or an alternate is noted in the ingredient listing, and this change will not affect the overall essence of the dish, it will not be highlighted. Notes about omissions or replacements that may change the dish more significantly will be noted in the shaded box (element 7).

4 Ingredients list.

5 Preparation instructions.

6 Additional recipe or prep photos.

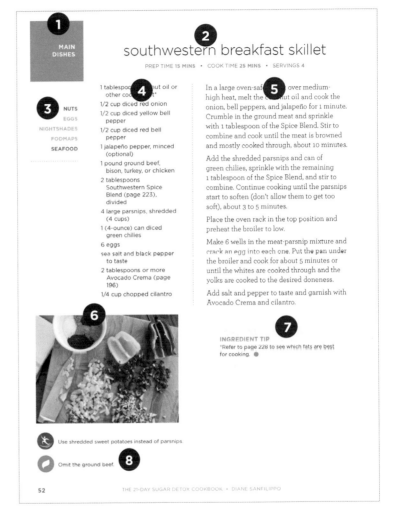

7 Special notes regarding where to find ingredients, special preparation techniques, ingredient swaps or omissions for allergens, and any other information that is relevant and important to note before prepping the recipe.

8 Modifications icons are shown without a note if the recipe is suitable for that modification as-written. Icons are shown with a note if an ingredient swap or omission will allow the recipe to be compliant. For example, in the above recipe swapping sweet potatoes for parsnips will allow this recipe to suit Energy Modifications and omitting the ground beef will allow it to suit Pescetarian Modifications. Remember that all recipes are suitable for all Levels of the program, but if you are following modifications, you should pay attention to these icons and any additional notes.

special ingredients
a breakdown of some of the common ingredients used in this book

ALMOND BUTTER

WHAT IS IT?
A thick paste made from ground almonds that is a replacement for peanut or cashew butter.

WHY USE IT?
The 21DSD program does not include peanuts or cashews.

HOW MUCH?
I recommend that you be judicious with your use of almond and other nut butters (walnut, pecan, hazelnut) while on The 21DSD. There is no set allowed amount, but you may find that you are overindulging and creating unwanted habits if you make too many almond butter-based items or do not serve yourself limited portions. The treat recipes in this book that are made with almond butter all note serving sizes.

ALMOND FLOUR

WHAT IS IT?
A replacement for wheat or other grain flours that acts almost identically to wheat flour in baking.

WHY USE IT?
The 21DSD program does not include any grain flours.

HOW MUCH?
I recommend that you be judicious with your use of almond and other nut flours while on The 21DSD. There is no set allowed amount, but you may find that you are overindulging and creating unwanted habits if you bake too many almond flour-based items. The treat recipes in this book that are made with almond flour all note serving sizes.

ALMOND MEAL

WHAT IS IT?
A replacement for wheat or other grain flour or meal that adds crunch or texture to recipes and is great for coating or "breading."

WHY USE IT?
The 21DSD program does not include any grain flours or meals.

HOW MUCH?
I recommend that you be judicious with your use of almond and other nut meals while on The 21DSD.

APPLE CIDER VINEGAR

WHAT IS IT?
A type of vinegar made by fermenting apples. Use it in dressings and sauces.

WHY USE IT?
It is naturally gluten-free and a natural digestive aid.

HOW MUCH?
There is no limit to how much apple cider vinegar you can use while on The 21DSD.

CLARIFIED BUTTER & GHEE

WHAT IS IT?
Pure butterfat that is made by cooking the dairy solids out of whole butter. Ghee is clarified butter taken one step further (see page 218 for details).

WHY USE IT?
It is more heat-stable than butter with dairy proteins intact.

HOW MUCH?
There is no limit to how much clarified butter and ghee you can use while on The 21DSD.

COCONUT AMINOS

WHAT IS IT?
A fermented coconut sap product. Use it as you would use soy sauce.

WHY USE IT?
Soy is not included on The 21DSD, and this is a soy-sauce replacement. It is gluten-free and contains less sodium than soy sauce.

HOW MUCH?
You can use coconut aminos fairly liberally.

COCONUT BUTTER

WHAT IS IT?
A nut butter-like product made from finely ground coconut meat.

WHY USE IT?
Coconut butter can be used in place of nut butter if you have a nut allergy, and it can add texture, fat, and flavor to many recipes.

HOW MUCH?
You may eat any amount of coconut butter you like each day, but more than 2 tablespoons will likely be overwhelming.

COCONUT FLOUR

WHAT IS IT?
A high-fiber flour made from very finely ground coconut meat.

WHY USE IT?
Grain flours are not included on The 21DSD. If you have a nut allergy or prefer not to use nut flours, coconut flour is a good option.

HOW MUCH?
I recommend using coconut flour judiciously. Understand that it cannot be subbed 1:1 in recipes that call for other flours. Coconut flour generally requires more eggs than other flours to yield a moist result due to its high fiber content.

COCONUT**MILK**

WHAT IS IT?
A nondairy milk that can be made from scratch (see page 210 for a recipe) or purchased in cans. I don't recommend the type sold in cartons due to the high number of additives they contain.

WHY USE IT?
If you are following a dairy-free way of eating, are lactose or casein intolerant, or are on Level 3 of The 21DSD, you may choose coconut milk. It is great in Asian recipes and adds flavor and fat to them.

HOW MUCH?
There is no set limit to how much coconut milk you can have while on The 21DSD, but I don't recommend more than about 8 ounces per day.

COCONUT**OIL**

WHAT IS IT?
A naturally occurring saturated fat that can be used in sweet or savory dishes.

WHY USE IT?
It is extremely heat-stable and is ideal for cooking at higher temperatures as well as in treat recipes.

HOW MUCH?
There is no limit to how much coconut oil you can use while on The 21DSD.

COLD-PRESSED SESAME OIL

WHAT IS IT?
Oil made from whole sesame seeds using a cold-pressing method.

WHY USE IT?
It adds a rich flavor to finish Asian dishes.

HOW MUCH?
There is no limit to how much sesame oil you can use while on The 21DSD.

EXTRA-VIRGIN OLIVE OIL

WHAT IS IT?
Olive oil made from the first pressing of the olives.

WHY USE IT?
It has an amazing richness and carries nutrients, including vitamin E and polyphenols.

HOW MUCH?
There is no limit to how much olive oil you can use while on The 21DSD.

FISH**SAUCE**

WHAT IS IT?
A sauce made from fish fermented with salt that is used in traditional Asian cooking.

WHY USE IT?
It adds great flavor and provides the base for the umami (pleasant savory taste) in Asian dishes.

HOW MUCH?
There is no limit to how much fish sauce you can use while on The 21DSD.

GELATIN

WHAT IS IT?
A powdered derivative of the collagen from animal bones, traditionally pig or cow.

WHY USE IT?
It binds ingredients together and, more importantly, is a rich source of dietary collagen, glycine, and protein.

HOW MUCH?
There is no limit to how much gelatin you can use while on The 21DSD.

SESAME**TAHINI**

WHAT IS IT?
A thick paste made from ground sesame seeds that is a replacement for peanut, cashew, or other nut/seed butters, primarily in savory dishes.

WHY USE IT?
If you have a nut allergy, you may find this seed-based option useful for snacks.

HOW MUCH?
I recommend that you be judicious with your use of seed butters while on The 21DSD. There is no set allowed amount.

SUNBUTTER

WHAT IS IT?
A thick paste made from ground sunflower seeds that is a replacement for peanut, cashew, and other nut butters.

WHY USE IT?
If you have a nut allergy, you may find this seed-based option useful for snacks.

HOW MUCH?
I recommend that you be judicious with your use of seed butters while on The 21DSD. There is no set allowed amount, but you may find that you are overindulging and creating unwanted habits if you make too many sunbutter-based items or do not limit portions. The treat recipes in this book that are made with sunbutter all note serving sizes.

SECTION 2

levels & **meal plans**

which level to follow

"Sugar leaves you stranded; I make sure I have the proper amount of protein before I work out." —Evander Holyfield

The 21-Day Sugar Detox has three main levels.

The differences between the levels and modifications for the various tracks, while minor at first glance, translate into some very different food choices on a daily basis. In order to determine which level you should follow, as well as any possible modifications you may want to make, complete this short self-quiz.

SELF-QUIZ

Select the answer that **best** describes you.

1. **Are you new to The 21-Day Sugar Detox?**
   a) yes
   b) no, I have completed it once
   c) no, I have completed it two or more times

2. **I currently eat:**
   a) bread, pasta, and other foods made from whole grain or other types of grain flour (wheat, teff, spelt, kamut, rye, etc.)
   b) bread, pasta, and other foods made from gluten-free grain flours
   c) a grain-free, Paleo, or primal type of diet

3. **I currently eat:**
   a) fat-free dairy products
   b) low-fat dairy products
   c) full-fat dairy products or no dairy

4. **I feel that my sugar and carb cravings are:**
   a) *so* strong that I'm admittedly fearful of how this detox will go for me
   b) pretty darned strong—that's why I'm reading this!
   c) not terrible, but certainly not under control the way I think they should be

5. **I:**
   a) am currently following a pescetarian diet—I eat seafood, eggs, and dairy, but not meat
   b) am currently pregnant or nursing
   c) live a very active lifestyle, work at a physically demanding job, or participate in high-intensity physical activity or exercise regularly
   d) have been diagnosed with an autoimmune condition
   e) none of the above

Results

QUESTIONS #1–4

Determines which level is right for you.

- If you answered mostly "a," then select **Level 1.**
- If you answered mostly "b," then select **Level 2.**
- If you answered mostly "c," then select **Level 3.**

QUESTION #5

Determines the modifications, if any, to the level you determined is right for you based on your answers to questions #1–4.

- If you answered "a," then follow the Pescetarian Modifications on page 27 (for Level 1) or page 35 (for Level 2).
- If you answered "b" or "c," then follow the Energy Modifications on page 26 (for Level 1), page 34 (for Level 2), or page 42 (for Level 3).
- If you answered "d," then follow the Autoimmune Modifications on page 43.
- If you answered "e," then simply follow the level that is right for you.

While Level 1 is the most lenient plan and Level 3 is the strictest, Level 1 will likely be your best bet if dietary changes are a new endeavor for you. That said, the level you tackle is *absolutely your choice.* You may find that Level 1 is a great choice for your first time through, and that returning to complete the program at Level 2 and then Level 3 will be quite effective and present different challenges and results.

THE MODIFICATIONS

The Pescetarian, Energy, and Autoimmune Modifications have been created to enhance your experience if you fall into one of those categories for nutritional needs. It's important that you follow the recommended modifications, as you will likely struggle with more severe detox symptoms. Each track has some specifications that are not necessarily aligned with every level. For example, the Pescetarian Modifications are not appropriate in combination with Level 3 food choices because that level omits many foods that pescetarians will need to rely on for nutrition.

• DON'T BE A HERO! •
An important note about selecting a level and following modifications

The levels and modifications were created and refined after thousands of people completed the program. Completing a higher level just to challenge yourself more is not necessarily going to yield a better result.

You can always come back for another round of The 21DSD at a different level or using different modifications, but use this self-quiz to best determine where to start each time! ●

Is it a "Yes" food?

While you follow the guidelines and Yes/No Foods Lists outlined in the following pages, you may encounter foods that are not listed, or you may be slightly confused about whether a particular food is included in or excluded from the program. Read the Yes/No Foods List for your level thoroughly, then follow these basic principles of The 21DSD to direct your choices and help you figure out whether or not you should eat the food in question.

- **Added sweeteners are not allowed.** The only way to enjoy a somewhat sweet taste is to use the included fruits in the limited portions as outlined in your Yes/No Foods List. If an added sweetener is included in the ingredients list of a packaged item you want to eat, it is not allowed. Note that some foods on your Yes list, such as full-fat dairy on Levels 1 and 2, contain natural sugars, and these are okay. Bacon that includes sugar in its ingredients is okay, as long as the total grams of carbs per serving does not exceed 1 gram.

- **If it tastes sweet and it isn't included on the Yes or Limit foods list for your level, it's not allowed.** Some herbal teas taste sweet naturally, and these are allowed. Otherwise, if an item tastes sweet and you aren't sure about it, leave it out.

- **Grain flours are not allowed.** This means you will not eat any foods made from whole-grain or refined-grain flours (wheat, spelt, and quinoa flours, for example). The only flours allowed are those made from nuts, seeds, coconut, or some limited starches (like tapioca or arrowroot flour when used as a thickening agent in sauces).

- **When in doubt, leave it out.** If you find it difficult to make a judgment call about a particular food on your own, login to the forums at balancedbites.com/21DSD to ask your question and get more answers and support.

TOP 10 SUGAR DETOX TIPS

1. **SLEEP.** If you're not getting enough sleep, you're setting yourself up for a full day's worth of cravings.

2. **DRINK WATER.** Stay hydrated to be sure that when you think you're feeling hungry, it's not actually thirst kicking in.

3. **BE PREPARED.** Having the right foods on hand will get you through the day so that you can do your best to avoid cravings but have good food available if they hit.

4. **ENLIST A FRIEND.** Or coworker, or family member...you get the idea. Completing this challenge with the support of someone you spend time with daily can help tons.

5. **LEARN TO LOVE HERBAL TEA.** You can drink herbal tea (caffeine-free) to your heart's content. It often feels like a treat, so you won't feel deprived if you have a craving.

6. **PROTEIN FIRST, THEN FAT, THEN VEGGIES.** That's how you build a plate, whether it's a meal or a snack.

7. **TURN MEALS INTO SNACKS.** Prepare just a little bit extra when you make a meal, and stash leftovers in a container for a snack if you need it. A snack doesn't need to be "snack food."

8. **TAKE A WALK.** When you feel like you want a sweet treat, a distraction or some physical activity can often get your mind refocused.

9. **REDUCE CAFFEINE.** Caffeine encourages your body to crave sugar. If you're struggling, work on reducing your caffeine intake over the first week.

10. **RELAX!** Stressing about the detox will only make you crave more sugar!

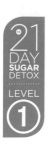

level 1

notes for level 1 that explain its differences from the other levels

While completing The 21-Day Sugar Detox at Level 1, you may choose to follow this meal plan to the letter, follow parts of it to suit your needs and tastes, or simply follow your Yes/No Foods List on pages 24–25 along with these general notes.

The following foods are optional to include with meals or snacks; you can leave them out if you choose on some days. *Optional items appear in* **bold italics** *in the meal plan.*

WHOLE GRAINS & LEGUMES
up to 1/2 cup total per day, cooked
Only gluten-free grains are included in this program.

- amaranth
- arrowroot
- beans: black, fava, navy, pinto, red
- buckwheat
- garbanzo beans (chickpeas)
- lentils
- millet
- quinoa
- rice (white, brown, wild)
- sorghum
- tapioca

Note that foods made *from* the included whole grains (for instance, brown rice pasta and whole-grain cereals) are *not* approved.

If you are following the meal plan provided here, I have added your 1/2 cup per day of grains or legumes to meals in the plan based on the cuisine types and flavor combinations.

If you are not following the meal plan specifically, you will need to add your 1/2 cup serving where you see fit. If you plan on cooking from the recipes in this book, they

are approved for *all* levels and do not include grains or legumes.

Feel free to adjust when you eat your portion. For example, if rice is planned at lunch but you generally feel better including your additional carbs at dinner, you can absolutely do that. In general, I find that including carbs later in the day leads to better sleep and more even blood sugar levels throughout the day.

FULL-FAT DAIRY *no specific portion limits*
Nonfat and low-fat dairy products are not allowed.

- cheese, cream cheese, cottage cheese
- whole milk, heavy cream, half & half
- plain, full-fat yogurt or kefir
- sour cream

You may choose to include full-fat dairy in your daily meal plan or just occasionally. There are some suggestions for where you may add it within the plan that follows. Choose local, grass-fed, and non-homogenized varieties whenever possible. Organic is recommended if you are unable to find grass-fed dairy.

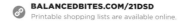
BALANCEDBITES.COM/21DSD
Printable shopping lists are available online.

MEAL PLAN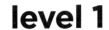

level 1

DAY	BREAKFAST	LUNCH	DINNER	SNACK
1 ● ▲ ■	worth-the-wait crustless quiche (54), steamed green vegetable*	[make ahead] jalapeño-dill tuna salad (110) with leafy greens salad or lettuce wraps	lamb burgers with chunky avo-ziki (102), beet & carrot stacked salad (135) or *1/2 cup quinoa*	[make ahead] turkey jerky (174) + choice of nuts or smoky lime nut mix (171) or *full-fat cheese*
2 ● ■ ▲	*leftover* worth-the-wait crustless quiche, steamed green vegetable*	*leftover* lamb burgers with chunky avo-ziki, *leftover* beet & carrot stacked salad or *1/2 cup quinoa*	no-honey mustard pecan-crusted salmon (116), mixed greens salad* & dressing^	*leftover* turkey jerky + *leftover* nut mix or *full-fat cheese*
3 ● ▲ ■ ◆	carrot-apple skillet breakfast hash (48)	*leftover* no-honey mustard pecan-crusted salmon, mixed greens salad* & dressing^	beef & bacon cottage pie (82), green salad* & dressing^ and *1/2 cup rice*	hard-boiled egg or *full-fat cheese* + salt & vinegar kale chips (172)
4 ● ■ ◆ ●	*leftover* carrot-apple skillet breakfast hash	*leftover* beef & bacon cottage pie, green salad* & dressing^	weeknight chicken soup (129), dill crackers (163), green vegetable* and *1/2 cup rice*	pesto deviled eggs (162) or *full-fat cheese* + *leftover* salt & vinegar kale chips
5 ● ● ●	smoothie of choice (49–51) with 2 eggs any style or 3oz protein of choice	*leftover* weeknight chicken soup, *leftover* dill crackers, green vegetable* and *1/2 cup rice*	artichoke & lemon chicken with capers (68), mixed greens salad* & dressing^	apple spice "granola" (178), full-fat milk of choice: **dairy**, coconut (210), or almond (212)
6 ● ● ▲	2 eggs any style or 3oz protein of choice with steamed green vegetables*	*leftover* artichoke & lemon chicken with capers, mixed greens salad* & dressing^	ahi tuna poke bowl (108) and *1/2 cup rice*	*leftover* apple spice "granola," *leftover* milk of choice
7 ● ▲ ◆	banana vanilla bean n'oatmeal (46)	green salad* & dressing^ with *leftover* protein of choice or canned wild salmon	coffee & cocoa rubbed ribs (100), spicy slaw (134) and *1/2 cup beans*	sundried tomato hummus (169), veggies

KEY
- ● Eggs
- ● Poultry
- ◆ Pork
- ■ Lamb
- ■ Beef/Bison
- ▲ Seafood

NOTES

*   choose any green vegetable from your Yes foods list on page 24

^   choose any of The 21DSD salad dressings

Add a starchy vegetable if you are following modifications that direct you to do so.

Bold italicized items are optional—you can add them or leave them out.

Icons denote the main protein source in meals for your planning purposes. Snacks are optional.

DAY	BREAKFAST	LUNCH	DINNER	SNACK
8 ● ◆ ●	*leftover* banana vanilla bean n'oatmeal	*leftover* coffee & cocoa rubbed ribs, spicy slaw (134), and **1/2 cup beans**	chicken strips (78), no-honey mustard sauce (202), roasted garlic parsnip mash (148), green salad*	*leftover* sundried tomato hummus, veggies
9 ● ● ■	pizza frittata (56)	*leftover* chicken strips, *leftover* no-honey mustard sauce, *leftover* roasted garlic parsnip mash, green salad*	satay skewers (94), broccoli double take (146), and **1/2 cup rice**	21DSD-friendly fruit + sunbutter (164) or nut butter or **full-fat cheese**
10 ● ■ ▲ ◆	*leftover* pizza frittata	*leftover* satay skewers, *leftover* broccoli double take and **1/2 cup rice**	cabbage-wrapped dumplings (120)	21DSD-friendly fruit + *leftover* sunbutter or **full-fat cheese**
11 ● ◆ ▲	smoothie of choice (49–51) with 2 eggs any style or 3oz protein of choice	[make ahead] cinnamon & fennel braised pork (84), roasted butternut squash mash (144), spiced applesauce (151)	salmon with creamy tzatziki sauce (114), creamy cucumber salad (152), green salad* and **1/2 cup quinoa**	apple spice "granola" (178), full-fat milk of choice: **dairy**, coconut (210), or almond (212)
12 ◆ ● ●	*leftover* cinnamon & fennel braised pork, *leftover* roasted butternut squash mash, *leftover* spiced applesauce	[make ahead] curried chicken salad with apples (80), carrot-ginger soup (126)	[make-ahead] slow cooker chicken adobo (70), creamy mushroom soup (132), and **1/2 cup beans**	*leftover* apple spice "granola," *leftover* milk of choice
13 ■ ● ● ●	southwestern breakfast skillet (52), avocado crema (196)	*leftover* curried chicken salad with apples, *leftover* carrot-ginger soup	bbq chicken (81), green bean casserole (154; *uses leftover* creamy mushroom soup), and **1/2 cup rice**	hard-boiled egg or **full-fat cheese** + salt & vinegar kale chips (172)
14 ● ● ◆	butternut squash pancakes (62), spiced buttery apple spread (203)	*leftover* bbq chicken, *leftover* green bean casserole, and **1/2 cup rice**	smoky grilled pork chops with cookout coleslaw (106), brussels sprouts with crispy capers & bacon (138)	pesto deviled eggs (162) or **full-fat cheese** + *leftover* salt & vinegar kale chips

KEY
● Eggs
● Poultry
◆ Pork
■ Lamb
■ Beef/Bison
▲ Seafood

NOTES
*   choose any green vegetable from your Yes foods list on page 24
^   choose any of The 21DSD salad dressings
Add a starchy vegetable if you are following modifications that direct you to do so.
Bold italicized items are optional—you can add them or leave them out.
Icons denote the main protein source in meals for planning purposes. Snacks are optional.

DAY	BREAKFAST	LUNCH	DINNER	SNACK
15 ● ◆ ▲	[make-ahead] nutty cinnamon crumb cake (182), 2 eggs any style or 3oz protein of choice	*leftover* smoky grilled pork chops with cookout coleslaw, *leftover* brussels sprouts with crispy capers & bacon	cilantro shrimp stir-fry (122), garlic & green onion cauli-rice (136) or *1/2 cup rice*	21DSD-friendly fruit + sunbutter (164) or nut butter or *full-fat cheese*
16 ● ◆ ■	*leftover* nutty cinnamon crumb cake, 2 eggs any style or 3oz protein of choice	[make-ahead] portuguese green soup (130) and *1/2 cup rice or beans*	chorizo burgers with spicy red onions (98), green salad* & dressing^	21DSD-friendly fruit + *leftover* sunbutter or nut butter or *full-fat cheese*
17 ● ◆ ●	mushroom & green onion frittata (58), avocado	*leftover* portuguese green soup	lemon ginger chicken (72), asian sautéed greens (140), and *1/2 cup rice*	apple spice "granola" (178), full-fat milk of choice: **dairy**, coconut (210), or almond (212)
18 ● ● ◆	smoothie of choice (49–51) with 2 eggs any style or 3oz protein of choice	*leftover* lemon ginger chicken, *leftover* asian sautéed greens, and *1/2 cup rice*	italian sausage & peppers (104), roasted garlic parsnip mash (148)	*leftover* apple spice "granola," *leftover* milk of choice
19 ● ◆ ●	smoothie of choice (49–51) with 2 eggs any style or 3oz protein of choice	*leftover* italian sausage & peppers, *leftover* roasted garlic parsnip mash	tandoori chicken skewers (74), moroccan cauli-rice pilaf (137) or *1/2 cup rice*	turkey jerky (174) + choice of nuts or smoky lime nut mix (171) or *full-fat cheese*
20 ● ◆ ● ■	[make-ahead] breakfast sausage & biscuit sandwich (60), steamed green vegetable*	*leftover* tandoori chicken skewers, *leftover* moroccan cauli-rice pilaf or *1/2 cup rice*	beef larb (thai lettuce wraps) (90)	*leftover* turkey jerky + *leftover* smoky lime nut mix or *full-fat cheese*
21 ● ■ ●	2 eggs any style or 3oz protein of choice with steamed green vegetables*	*leftover* beef larb (thai lettuce wraps)	chicken pot pie (66), mixed greens salad* & dressing^ and *1/2 cup rice*	sundried tomato hummus (169), veggies

KEY
- Eggs
- Poultry
- ◆ Pork
- ■ Lamb
- ■ Beef/Bison
- ▲ Seafood

NOTES

*   choose any green vegetable from your Yes foods list on page 24

^   choose any of The 21DSD salad dressings

Add a starchy vegetable if you are following modifications that direct you to do so.

Bold italicized items are optional—you can add them or leave them out.

Icons denote the main protein source in meals for planning purposes. Snacks are optional.

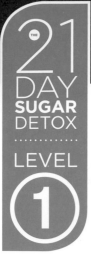

the yes / no foods list

THE 21 DAY SUGAR DETOX
LEVEL 1

DON'T SEE THE FOOD YOU WANT TO EAT ON THE LIST?

Review "Is it a Yes food?" on page 19.

MODIFICATIONS

If you are following the Energy or Pescetarian tracks, see the meal plan modifications on pages 26–27 for additional notes.

YES FOODS *eat plenty of these foods for 21 days*

MEAT, FISH, & EGGS
including but not limited to:
ALL meats, including deli and cured meats like bacon, pancetta, prosciutto, etc. (see page 226 for the best brands)
ALL seafood
Eggs

VEGETABLES
Artichokes/sunchokes
Asparagus
Broccoli
Brussels sprouts
Cabbage
Carrots
Cauliflower
Celery/celery root
Chard
Collards
Cucumber
Eggplant
Garlic
Ginger
Green beans
Horseradish
Jicama
Kale
Leeks
Lettuce, *all leafy greens*
Mushrooms
Onions
Parsnips
Peppers, *all varieties*
Radicchio
Radishes
Rutabaga
Snow/snap peas
Spaghetti squash
Spinach
Tomato
Turnips
Yellow squash
Zucchini

FRUIT
review the Limit foods for more fruit choices!
Lemon
Lime

NUTS/SEEDS
whole, flour, or butters
Almonds
Brazil nuts
Cocoa/cacao (100%), nibs
Chia seeds
Coconut, *all unsweetened forms are okay—coconut sugar is a NO*
Filberts (hazelnuts)
Flaxseed
Hemp seeds
Macadamia nuts
Pecans
Pistachios
Pumpkin seeds
Sunflower seeds
Sesame seeds, tahini
Walnuts

FATS & OILS
review the guide on page 228
Animal fats
Butter, ghee, clarified butter
Avocados, avocado oil
Coconut oil
Flax oil
Olives, olive oil
Sesame oil

DAIRY
full-fat only!
Cheese, cream cheese, cottage cheese
Milk, whole only
Half & half
Heavy cream
Sour cream
Yogurt/kefir, plain

BEVERAGES
Almond milk, unsweetened/homemade (page 212)
Coconut milk, coconut cream, full-fat
Coffee, espresso
Mineral water
Seltzer, club soda
Teas: herbal, green, black, white, etc., unsweetened
Water

CONDIMENTS/MISC.
Broth, homemade only (recipe on page 208)
Coconut aminos
Sweetener-Free Ketchup (recipe on page 216) *no store-bought ketchups are allowed*
Extracts: vanilla, almond, vanilla bean, etc.
Hummus made from cauliflower (recipe on page 169)
Healthy Homemade Mayonnaise (recipe on page 219) *do your best to avoid others*
Mustard, gluten-free varieties
Nutritional/Brewer's yeast (Lewis Labs brand)
Salad dressings, homemade
Spices & herbs: all are OK; check pre-mixed blends for hidden ingredients
Vinegars: apple cider, balsamic, distilled, red wine, rice, sherry, white

SUPPLEMENTS
Protein powder, 100% pure with NO other ingredients (e.g., 100% whey, egg white, or hemp)
Fermented cod liver oil, with or without flavor (one exception to the no-sweetener rule!)
Pure vitamin or mineral supplements

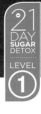

LIMIT FOODS *these are Yes foods with portion size limits*

VEGETABLES & STARCHES
1 cup serving per day is allowed
Acorn squash
Beets
Butternut squash
Green peas
Pumpkin
Winter squash (assorted)

FRUIT
1 piece per day is allowed
Bananas, green-tipped/
 not quite ripe only
Grapefruit
Green/Granny Smith
 apples

GRAINS/LEGUMES
*1/2 cup serving per day
(cooked) is allowed of whole
forms only—NO FLOURS*
Amaranth
Arrowroot
Beans: black, fava,
 garbanzo (chickpeas),
 navy, pinto, red
Buckwheat
Lentils
Millet
Quinoa
Rice (brown, white, wild)
Sorghum

BEVERAGES
1 cup total per day is allowed
Coconut juice, coco-
 nut water: (no added
 sweeteners)
Kombucha, home-
 brewed or store-bought
 (see recommended
 brands on page 226)

NO FOODS *do not eat these foods for 21 days*

REFINED CARBOHYDRATES
Bagels
Bread
Breadsticks
Brownies
Cake
Candy
Cereal/granola
Chips
Cookies
Couscous
Crackers
Croissants
Cupcakes
Muffins
Oats
Orzo
Pasta
Pastries
Pita
Pizza
Popcorn
Rice cakes
Rolls
Tortillas, tortilla chips

VEGETABLES & STARCHES
Cassava
Corn, polenta, grits
Plantains
Soybeans/edamame
Sweet potatoes/yams
Tapioca, whole & flour
Taro

FRUITS
*review the Yes and Limit foods
lists for included fruits*
Fresh & dried

GRAINS/LEGUMES
Barley
Kamut
Rye
Soybeans/edamame
 (including miso, natto,
 tempeh, tofu, and soy
 sauce)
Spelt
Wheat
Flours made from grains
 or beans (chickpeas,
 lentils, etc.)

NUTS/NUT BUTTERS
Cashew
Peanut

SWEETENERS OF ANY KIND
None are allowed!

ANYTHING "DIET," SUGAR-FREE, OR ARTIFICIALLY SWEETENED
This means no gum,
either!

SUPPLEMENTS
Anything that includes
 sugar, sweeteners, or
 sugar alcohols (xylitol,
 for example)
Shakeology and other
 similar blends
Supplements that con-
 tain soy, corn, or wheat

BEVERAGES
All alcohol
Coffee "drinks" or shakes,
 presweetened
Juice
Milk: skim, nonfat, 1%, 2%,
 soy/rice/oat
Soda (regular & diet)
Sweet-tasting drinks
 (besides herbal teas)
Protein powders that
 have more than one
 ingredient (see Yes food
 supplements)

CONDIMENTS/MISC.
Broth/stock in a box/can
Hummus made from
 garbanzo beans
Ketchup, store-bought
Mayonnaise, store-bought
Salad dressings, pre-
 made/store-bought
Soy sauce, tamari

additional notes for those who need more carbohydrates

THESE MODIFICATIONS MAY BE RIGHT FOR YOU IF YOU
· live a very active lifestyle or work at a physically demanding job
· participate in high-intensity physical activity or exercise regularly (for example, interval training, CrossFit-style workouts, endurance athletics, or cardio/aerobic activity at moderate to high intensity for more than 20 minutes at a time; yoga alone doesn't typically require these modifications)
· are pregnant or nursing

With the Energy Modifications, your portion of whole grains or legumes will increase. You will also need to add to your meal plan starchy carbohydrate vegetables that are considered No foods for those who do not fit the modification requirements listed above.

WHOLE GRAINS & LEGUMES
include up to 1 cup total per day, cooked
As noted under the Limit foods on your Yes/No Foods List.

STARCHY CARBOHYDRATE VEGETABLES
amount varies based on your activity level and energy requirements; see page 230 for a list of these foods
Add 30–50 grams of carbohydrates to a *minimum* of one meal per day, especially after exercise. This means 1/2 to 1 cup of mashed sweet potato, for example. You should also use the one piece of fruit per day included for all Level 1 detoxers to reach this carbohydrate goal.

If you train very hard (at high intensity or more than once a day), you may need to make this modification for *each instance* of exercise—meaning more than one meal or snack will include up to 30–50 grams of dense carbohydrates.

You may adjust when you eat your extra carbs. For example, if sweet potato is listed at lunch but you generally feel better including your additional carbs at dinner, you can absolutely do that. In general, adding more carbs later in the day or after activity tends to replenish your fuel better. *This is a highly variable element in your meal planning, and tracking your own energy levels is the best way to decide when to consume your extra carbs.*

RECOMMENDED CARBS PER DAY
Moderately active: 75–150 grams
Highly active: 100–200+ grams
Pregnant/nursing: 100+ grams
These are estimates. If you find that you need more carbs to maintain activity, adjust to your needs.

If you are pregnant or nursing, add these carbohydrate sources as you see fit. Do not limit them assuming it will lead to better results. The goal of this program is a healthy body and a healthy baby, and limiting these foods further is absolutely not necessary! If you find that your milk supply is low or you feel more fatigued than usual, increase your intake of more carbohydrate-dense foods as outlined here.

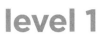
additional notes for those who eat
seafood, eggs, and dairy, but not meat

THESE MODIFICATIONS MAY BE RIGHT FOR YOU IF YOU

· follow a pescetarian diet

With the Pescetarian Modifications, your portion of whole grains or legumes will increase. You will also need to add to your meal plan starchy carbohydrate vegetables that are considered No foods for those who do not fit the modification requirements listed above.

WHOLE GRAINS & LEGUMES
you may include up to 1 cup per day total, cooked

As noted under the Limit foods on your Yes/No Foods List. It is not required that you eat the approved grains or legumes every day if you are eating sufficient amounts of other protein and carb sources.

STARCHY CARBOHYDRATE VEGETABLES
see page 230 for a list of these foods

FULL-FAT DAIRY *no specific portion limits*

You may want to add some high-quality dairy to meals for additional protein and fat. Choose local, grass-fed, and non-homogenized varieties whenever possible. Organic is recommended if you are unable to find grass-fed dairy.

EXTRA FATS
add extra fat portions to meals and snacks

For example:

· add a whole avocado to a meal instead of a half
· add 1/4 cup nuts and/or dressing to a salad instead of 2 tablespoons
· make good use of full-fat dairy products for fat and protein if you tolerate dairy well (tolerating dairy means that you don't experience symptoms such as gas, bloating, digestive distress, acne, eczema, or congestion when you eat it)

SEAFOOD
make seafood your protein source in at least one meal per day, ideally two

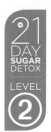

level 2

notes for level 2 that explain its differences from the other levels

While completing The 21-Day Sugar Detox at Level 2, you may choose to follow this meal plan to the letter, follow parts of it to suit your needs or tastes, or simply follow your Yes/No Foods List on pages 32–33 along with these general notes.

The following foods are optional to include with meals or snacks; you can leave them out if you choose on some days. *Optional items appear in **bold italics** in the meal plan.*

FULL-FAT DAIRY
no specific portion limits
Nonfat or low-fat dairy products are not allowed.

- cheese, cream cheese, cottage cheese
- whole milk, heavy cream, half & half
- plain, full-fat yogurt or kefir
- sour cream

You may choose to include full-fat dairy in your daily meal plan or just occasionally. There are some suggestions of where you may add it within the plan that follows. Choose local, grass-fed, and non-homogenized varieties whenever possible. Organic is recommended if you are unable to find grass-fed dairy.

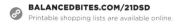

BALANCEDBITES.COM/21DSD
Printable shopping lists are available online.

level 2

DAY	BREAKFAST	LUNCH	DINNER	SNACK
1 ● ▲ ■	worth-the-wait crustless quiche (54), steamed green vegetable*	[make ahead] jalapeño-dill tuna salad (110) with leafy greens salad or lettuce wraps	lamb burgers with chunky avo-ziki (102), beet & carrot stacked salad (135)	[make ahead] turkey jerky (174) + choice of nuts or smoky lime nut mix (171) or *full-fat cheese*
2 ● ■ ▲	*leftover* worth-the-wait crustless quiche, steamed green vegetable*	*leftover* lamb burgers with chunky avo-ziki, *leftover* beet & carrot stacked salad	no-honey mustard pecan-crusted salmon (116), mixed greens salad* & dressing^	*leftover* turkey jerky + *leftover* nut mix or *full-fat cheese*
3 ● ▲ ■ ◆	carrot-apple skillet breakfast hash (48)	*leftover* no-honey mustard pecan-crusted salmon, mixed greens salad* & dressing^	beef & bacon cottage pie (82), green salad* & dressing^	hard-boiled egg or *full-fat cheese* + salt & vinegar kale chips (172)
4 ● ■ ◆ ●	*leftover* carrot-apple skillet breakfast hash	*leftover* beef & bacon cottage pie, green salad* & dressing^	weeknight chicken soup (129), dill crackers (163), green vegetable*	pesto deviled eggs (162) or *full-fat cheese* + *leftover* salt & vinegar kale chips
5 ● ● ●	smoothie of choice (49–51) with 2 eggs any style or 3oz protein of choice	*leftover* weeknight chicken soup, *leftover* dill crackers, green vegetable*	artichoke & lemon chicken with capers (68), mixed greens salad* & dressing^	apple spice "granola" (178), full-fat milk of choice: *dairy*, coconut (210), or almond (212)
6 ● ● ▲	2 eggs any style or 3oz protein of choice with steamed green vegetables*	*leftover* artichoke & lemon chicken with capers, mixed greens salad* & dressing^	ahi tuna poke bowl (108)	*leftover* apple spice "granola," *leftover* milk of choice
7 ● ▲ ◆	banana vanilla bean chia n'oatmeal (46)	green salad* & dressing^ with *leftover* protein of choice or canned wild salmon	coffee & cocoa rubbed ribs (100), spicy slaw (134)	sundried tomato hummus (169), veggies

KEY
- ● Eggs
- ● Poultry
- ◆ Pork
- ■ Lamb
- ■ Beef/Bison
- ▲ Seafood

NOTES

*   choose any green vegetable from your Yes foods list on page 32

^   choose any of The 21DSD salad dressings

Add a starchy vegetable if you are following modifications that direct you to do so.

Bold italicized items are optional—you can add them or leave them out.

Icons denote the main protein source in meals for planning purposes. Snacks are optional.

level 2

DAY	BREAKFAST	LUNCH	DINNER	SNACK
8 ● ◆ ●	*leftover* banana vanilla bean n'oatmeal	*leftover* coffee & cocoa rubbed ribs, *leftover* spicy slaw	chicken strips (78), no-honey mustard sauce (202), roasted garlic parsnip mash (148), green salad*	*leftover* sundried tomato hummus, veggies
9 ● ● ■	pizza frittata (56)	*leftover* chicken strips, *leftover* no-honey mustard sauce, *leftover* roasted garlic parsnip mash, green salad*	satay skewers (94), broccoli double take (146)	21DSD-friendly fruit + sunbutter (164) or nut butter or ***full-fat cheese***
10 ● ■ ▲ ◆	*leftover* pizza frittata	*leftover* satay skewers, *leftover* broccoli double take	cabbage-wrapped dumplings (120)	21DSD-friendly fruit + *leftover* sunbutter or ***full-fat cheese***
11 ● ◆ ▲	smoothie of choice (49–51) with 2 eggs any style or 3oz protein of choice	[make ahead] cinnamon & fennel braised pork (84), roasted butternut squash mash (144), spiced applesauce (151)	salmon with creamy tzatziki sauce (114), creamy cucumber salad (152), green salad* & dressing^	apple spice "granola" (178), full-fat milk of choice: **dairy**, coconut (210), or almond (212)
12 ◆ ● ●	*leftover* cinnamon & fennel braised pork, *leftover* roasted butternut squash mash, *leftover* spiced applesauce	[make ahead] curried chicken salad with apples (80), carrot-ginger soup (126)	[make-ahead] slow cooker chicken adobo (70), creamy mushroom soup (132)	*leftover* apple spice "granola," *leftover* milk of choice
13 ■ ● ● ●	southwestern breakfast skillet (52), avocado crema (196)	*leftover* curried chicken salad with apples, *leftover* carrot-ginger soup	bbq chicken (81), green bean casserole (154; uses *leftover* creamy mushroom soup)	hard-boiled egg or ***full-fat cheese*** + salt & vinegar kale chips (172)
14 ● ● ◆	butternut squash pancakes (62), spiced buttery apple spread (203)	*leftover* bbq chicken, *leftover* green bean casserole	smoky grilled pork chops with cookout coleslaw (106), brussels sprouts with crispy capers & bacon (138)	pesto deviled eggs (162) or ***full-fat cheese*** + *leftover* salt & vinegar kale chips

KEY
- ● Eggs
- ● Poultry
- ◆ Pork
- ■ Lamb
- ■ Beef/Bison
- ▲ Seafood

NOTES
*   choose any green vegetable from your Yes foods list on page 33
^   choose any of The 21DSD salad dressings
Add a starchy vegetable if you are following modifications that direct you to do so.
Bold italicized items are optional—you can add them or leave them out.
Icons denote the main protein source in meals for planning purposes. Snacks are optional.

MEAL PLAN

level 2

DAY	BREAKFAST	LUNCH	DINNER	SNACK
15 ● ◆ ▲	[make-ahead] nutty cinnamon crumb cake (182), 2 eggs any style or 3oz protein of choice	*leftover* smoky grilled pork chops with cookout coleslaw, *leftover* brussels sprouts with crispy capers & bacon	cilantro shrimp stir-fry (122), garlic & green onion cauli-rice (136)	21DSD-friendly fruit + sunbutter (164) or nut butter or ***full-fat cheese***
16 ● ◆ ■	*leftover* nutty cinnamon crumb cake, 2 eggs any style or 3oz protein of choice	[make-ahead] portuguese green soup (130)	chorizo burgers with spicy red onions (98), green salad* & dressing^	21DSD-friendly fruit + *leftover* sunbutter or nut butter or ***full-fat cheese***
17 ● ● ●	mushroom & green onion frittata (58), avocado	*leftover* portuguese green soup	lemon ginger chicken (72), asian sautéed greens (140)	apple spice "granola" (178), full-fat milk of choice: ***dairy***, coconut (210), or almond (212)
18 ● ● ◆	smoothie of choice (49–51) with 2 eggs any style or 3oz protein of choice	*leftover* lemon ginger chicken, *leftover* asian sautéed greens	italian sausage & peppers (104), roasted garlic parsnip mash (148)	*leftover* apple spice "granola," *leftover* milk of choice
19 ● ● ●	smoothie of choice (49–51) with 2 eggs any style or 3oz protein of choice	*leftover* italian sausage & peppers, *leftover* roasted garlic parsnip mash	tandoori chicken skewers (74), moroccan cauli-rice pilaf (137)	turkey jerky (174) + choice of nuts or smoky lime nut mix (171) or ***full-fat cheese***
20 ● ◆ ● ■	[make-ahead] breakfast sausage & biscuit sandwich (60), steamed green vegetable*	*leftover* tandoori chicken skewers, *leftover* moroccan cauli-rice pilaf	beef larb (thai lettuce wraps) (90)	*leftover* turkey jerky + *leftover* smoky lime nut mix or ***full-fat cheese***
21 ● ■ ●	2 eggs any style or 3oz protein of choice with steamed green vegetables*	*leftover* beef larb (thai lettuce wraps)	chicken pot pie (66), mixed greens salad* & dressing^	sundried tomato hummus (169), veggies

KEY
● Eggs
● Poultry
◆ Pork
■ Lamb
■ Beef/Bison
▲ Seafood

NOTES
*   choose any green vegetable from your Yes foods list on page 33
^   choose any of The 21DSD salad dressings
Add a starchy vegetable if you are following modifications that direct you to do so.
Bold italicized items are optional—you can add them or leave them out.
Icons denote the main protein source in meals for planning purposes. Snacks are optional.

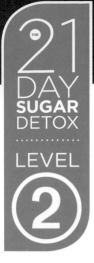

THE 21 DAY SUGAR DETOX

LEVEL 2

DON'T SEE THE FOOD YOU WANT TO EAT ON THE LIST?
Review "Is it a Yes food?" on page 19.

MODIFICATIONS
If you are following the Energy or Pescetarian tracks, see the meal plan modifications on pages 34-35 for additional notes.

YES FOODS *eat plenty of these foods for 21 days*

MEAT, FISH, & EGGS
including but not limited to:
ALL meats, including deli and cured meats like bacon, pancetta, prosciutto, etc. (see page 226 for the best brands)
ALL seafood
Eggs

VEGETABLES
Artichokes/sunchokes
Asparagus
Broccoli
Brussels sprouts
Cabbage
Carrots
Cauliflower
Celery/celery root
Chard
Collards
Cucumber
Eggplant
Garlic
Ginger
Green beans
Horseradish
Jicama
Kale
Leeks
Lettuce, *all leafy greens*
Mushrooms
Onions
Parsnips
Peppers, *all varieties*
Radicchio
Radishes
Rutabaga
Snow/snap peas
Spaghetti squash
Spinach
Tomato
Turnips
Yellow squash
Zucchini

FRUIT
review the Limit foods for more fruit choices!
Lemon
Lime

NUTS/SEEDS
whole, flour, or butters
Almonds
Brazil nuts
Cocoa/cacao (100%), nibs
Chia seeds
Coconut, *all unsweetened forms are okay—coconut sugar is a NO*
Filberts (hazelnuts)
Flaxseed
Hemp seeds
Macadamia nuts
Pecans
Pistachios
Pumpkin seeds
Sunflower seeds
Sesame seeds, tahini
Walnuts

FATS & OILS
review the guide on page 228
Animal fats
Butter, ghee, clarified butter
Avocados, avocado oil
Coconut oil
Flax oil
Olives, olive oil
Sesame oil

DAIRY
full-fat only!
Cheese, cream cheese, cottage cheese
Milk, whole only
Half & half
Heavy cream
Sour cream
Yogurt/kefir, plain

BEVERAGES
Almond milk, unsweetened/homemade (page 212)
Coconut milk, coconut cream, full-fat
Coffee, espresso
Mineral water
Seltzer, club soda
Teas: herbal, green, black, white, etc., unsweetened
Water

CONDIMENTS/MISC.
Broth, homemade only (recipe on page 208)
Coconut aminos
Sweetener-Free Ketchup (recipe on page 216) *no store-bought ketchups are allowed*
Extracts: vanilla, almond, vanilla bean, etc.
Hummus made from cauliflower (recipe on page 169)
Healthy Homemade Mayonnaise (recipe on page 219) *do your best to avoid others*
Mustard, gluten-free varieties
Nutritional/Brewer's yeast (Lewis Labs brand)
Salad dressings, homemade
Spices & herbs: all are OK; check premixed blends for hidden ingredients
Vinegars: apple cider, balsamic, distilled, red wine, rice, sherry, white

SUPPLEMENTS
Protein powder, 100% pure with NO other ingredients (e.g., 100% whey, egg white, or hemp)
Fermented cod liver oil, with or without flavor (one exception to the no-sweetener rule!)
Pure vitamin or mineral supplements

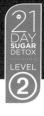

LIMIT FOODS *these are Yes foods with portion size limits*

VEGETABLES & STARCHES
1 cup serving per day is allowed
Acorn squash
Beets
Butternut squash
Green peas
Pumpkin
Winter squash (assorted)

FRUIT
1 piece per day is allowed
Bananas, green-tipped/
   not quite ripe only
Grapefruit
Green/Granny Smith
   apples

BEVERAGES
1 cup total per day is allowed
Coconut juice, coconut
   water (no added sweet-
   eners)
Kombucha, home-
   brewed or store-bought
   (see recommended
   brands on page 226)

NO FOODS *do not eat these foods for 21 days*

REFINED CARBOHYDRATES
Bagels
Bread
Breadsticks
Brownies
Cake
Candy
Cereal/granola
Chips
Cookies
Couscous
Crackers
Croissants
Cupcakes
Muffins
Oats
Orzo
Pasta
Pastries
Pita
Pizza
Popcorn
Rice cakes
Rolls
Tortillas, tortilla chips

VEGETABLES & STARCHES
Cassava
Corn, polenta, grits
Plantains
Soybeans/edamame
Sweet potatoes/yams
Tapioca, whole & flour
Taro

FRUITS
*review the Yes and Limit foods
lists for included fruits*
Fresh & dried

GRAINS/LEGUMES
Amaranth
Arrowroot
Barley
Beans: black, fava,
   garbanzo (chickpeas),
   navy, pinto, red
Buckwheat
Flours made from grains
   or beans (chickpeas,
   lentils, etc.)
Kamut
Lentils
Millet
Quinoa
Rice (brown, white, wild)
Rye
Sorghum
Soybeans/edamame
   (including miso, natto,
   tempeh, tofu, and soy
   sauce)
Spelt
Wheat

NUTS/NUT BUTTERS
Cashew
Peanut

SWEETENERS OF ANY KIND
None are allowed!

ANYTHING "DIET," SUGAR-FREE, OR ARTIFICIALLY SWEETENED
This means no gum,
either!

SUPPLEMENTS
Anything that includes
   sugar, sweeteners, or
   sugar alcohols (xylitol,
   for example)
Shakeology and other
   similar blends
Supplements that con-
   tain soy, corn, or wheat

BEVERAGES
All alcohol
Coffee "drinks" or shakes,
   presweetened
Juice
Milk: skim, nonfat, 1%, 2%,
   soy/rice/oat
Soda (regular & diet)
Sweet-tasting drinks
   (besides herbal teas)
Protein powders that
   have more than one
   ingredient (see Yes food
   supplements)

CONDIMENTS/MISC.
Broth/stock in a box/can
Hummus made from
   garbanzo beans
Ketchup, store-bought
Mayonnaise, store-bought
Salad dressings, pre-
   made/store-bought
Soy sauce, tamari

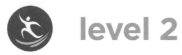

additional notes for those who need more carbohydrates

THESE MODIFICATIONS MAY BE RIGHT FOR YOU IF YOU

· live a very active lifestyle or work at a physically demanding job
· participate in high-intensity physical activity or exercise regularly (for example, interval training, CrossFit-style workouts, endurance athletics, or cardio/aerobic activity at moderate to high intensity for more than 20 minutes at a time; yoga alone doesn't typically require these modifications)
· are pregnant or nursing

With the Energy Modifications, you will need to add to your meal plan starchy carbohydrate vegetables that are considered No foods for those who do not fit the modification requirements listed above.

STARCHY CARBOHYDRATE VEGETABLES
amount varies based on your activity level and energy requirements; see page 230 for a list of these foods
Add 30–50 grams of carbohydrates to a *minimum* of one meal per day, especially after exercise. This means 1/2 to 1 cup of mashed sweet potato or plantain, for example. You should also use the one piece of fruit per day included for all Level 2 detoxers to reach this carbohydrate goal.

If you train very hard (at high intensity or more than once a day), you may need to make this modification for *each instance* of exercise—meaning more than one meal or snack will include up to this amount of dense carbohydrates.

You may adjust when you eat your extra carbs. For example, if sweet potato is listed at lunch but you generally feel better including your additional carbs at dinner, you can absolutely do that. In general, adding more carbs later in the day or after activity tends to replenish your fuel better. *This is a highly variable element in your meal planning, and tracking your own energy levels is the best way to decide when to consume your extra carbs.*

RECOMMENDED CARBS PER DAY
Moderately active: 75–150 grams
Highly active: 100–200+ grams
Pregnant/nursing: 100+ grams
These are estimates. If you find that you need more carbs to maintain activity, adjust to your needs.

If you are pregnant or nursing, add these carbohydrate sources as you see fit. Do not limit them assuming it will lead to better results. The goal of this program is a healthy body and a healthy baby, and limiting these foods further is absolutely not necessary! If you find that your milk supply is low or you feel more fatigued than usual, increase your intake of more carbohydrate-dense foods as outlined here.

*additional notes for those who eat
seafood, eggs, and dairy, but not meat*

THESE MODIFICATIONS MAY BE RIGHT FOR YOU IF YOU
· follow a pescetarian diet

With the Pescetarian Modifications, your portion of whole grains or legumes will increase. You will also need to add starchy carbohydrate vegetables to your meal plan that are considered No foods for those who do not fit the modification requirements listed above.

STARCHY CARBOHYDRATE VEGETABLES
*you may include up to 2 cups per day; see page 230 for
a list of these foods*

FULL-FAT DAIRY *no specific portion limits*
You may want to add some high-quality dairy to meals for additional protein and fat. Choose local, grass-fed, and non homogenized varieties whenever possible. Organic is recommended if you are unable to find grass-fed dairy.

EXTRA FATS
add extra fat portions to meals and snacks
For example:
· add a whole avocado to a meal instead of a half
· add 1/4 cup nuts and/or dressing to a salad instead of 2 tablespoons
· make good use of full-fat dairy products for fat and protein if you tolerate dairy well (tolerating dairy means that you don't experience symptoms such as gas, bloating, digestive distress, acne, eczema, or congestion when you eat it)

SEAFOOD
*make seafood your protein source for at least one
meal per day, ideally two*

level 3

notes for level 3 that explain its differences from the other levels

While completing The 21-Day Sugar Detox at Level 3, you may choose to follow this meal plan to the letter, follow parts of it to suit your needs or tastes, or simply follow your Yes/No Foods List on pages 40–41 along with these general notes.

This level is the most limited in terms of food choices. That said, Level 3 is not recommended simply because you may want to do the "hardest" or "strictest" level of the program. You should have landed here because your answers to the quiz on page 17 determined that this is the right plan for you.

What's different about Level 3 that sets it apart from Levels 1 and 2?
Level 3 excludes all grains and all dairy. This is often referred to as a Paleo type of diet. If you've read my book *Practical Paleo*, then you're familiar with this approach to nutrition. What The 21DSD does that's different from a standard Paleo approach is to remove excess natural sugars and sweet-tasting foods in order to change your habits around sweets and other foods that you rely on habitually.

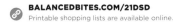

BALANCEDBITES.COM/21DSD
Printable shopping lists are available online.

level 3

DAY	BREAKFAST	LUNCH	DINNER	SNACK
1 ● ▲ ■	worth-the-wait crustless quiche (54), steamed green vegetable*	[make ahead] jalapeño-dill tuna salad (110) with leafy greens salad or lettuce wraps	lamb burgers with chunky avo-ziki (102), beet & carrot stacked salad (135)	[make ahead] turkey jerky (174) + choice of nuts or smoky lime nut mix (171)
2 ● ■ ▲	*leftover* worth-the-wait crustless quiche, steamed green vegetable*	*leftover* lamb burgers with chunky avo-ziki, *leftover* beet & carrot stacked salad	no-honey mustard pecan-crusted salmon (116), mixed greens salad* & dressing^	*leftover* turkey jerky + *leftover* nut mix
3 ● ▲ ■ ◆	carrot-apple skillet breakfast hash (48)	*leftover* no-honey mustard pecan-crusted salmon, mixed greens salad* & dressing^	beef & bacon cottage pie (82), green salad* & dressing^	hard-boiled egg + salt & vinegar kale chips (172)
4 ● ■ ◆ ●	*leftover* carrot-apple skillet breakfast hash	*leftover* beef & bacon cottage pie, green salad* & dressing^	weeknight chicken soup (129), dill crackers (163), green vegetable*	pesto deviled eggs (162) + *leftover* salt & vinegar kale chips
5 ● ● ●	smoothie of choice (49–51) with 2 eggs any style or 3oz protein of choice	*leftover* weeknight chicken soup, *leftover* dill crackers, green vegetable*	artichoke & lemon chicken with capers (68), mixed greens salad* & dressing^	apple spice "granola" (178), coconut (210) or almond milk (212)
6 ● ● ▲	2 eggs any style or 3oz protein of choice with steamed green vegetables*	*leftover* artichoke & lemon chicken with capers, mixed greens salad* & dressing^	ahi tuna poke bowl (108)	*leftover* apple spice "granola," *leftover* coconut or almond milk
7 ● ▲ ◆	banana vanilla bean n'oatmeal (46)	green salad* & dressing^ with *leftover* protein of choice or canned wild salmon	coffee & cocoa rubbed ribs (100), spicy slaw (134)	sundried tomato hummus (169), veggies

KEY
- ● Eggs
- ● Poultry
- ◆ Pork
- ■ Lamb
- ■ Beef/Bison
- ▲ Seafood

NOTES

*   choose any green vegetable from your Yes foods list on page 40

^   choose any of The 21DSD salad dressings

Add a starchy vegetable if you are following modifications that direct you to do so.

Bold italicized items are optional—you can add them or leave them out.

Icons denote the main protein source in meals for planning purposes. Snacks are optional.

level 3

DAY	BREAKFAST	LUNCH	DINNER	SNACK
8 ● ◆ ●	*leftover* banana vanilla bean n'oatmeal	*leftover* coffee & cocoa rubbed ribs, *leftover* spicy slaw	chicken strips (78), no-honey mustard sauce (202), roasted garlic parsnip mash (148), green salad*	*leftover* sundried tomato hummus, veggies
9 ● ● ■	pizza frittata (56)	*leftover* chicken strips, *leftover* no-honey mustard sauce, *leftover* roasted garlic parsnip mash, green salad*	satay skewers (94), broccoli double take (146)	21DSD-friendly fruit + sunbutter (164) or nut butter
10 ● ■ ▲ ◆	*leftover* pizza frittata	*leftover* satay skewers, *leftover* broccoli double take	cabbage-wrapped dumplings (120)	21DSD-friendly fruit + *leftover* sunbutter
11 ● ◆ ▲	smoothie of choice (49–51) with 2 eggs any style or 3oz protein of choice	[make ahead] cinnamon & fennel braised pork (84), roasted butternut squash mash (144), spiced applesauce (151)	salmon with creamy tzatziki sauce (114), creamy cucumber salad (152), green salad*	apple spice "granola" (178), coconut (210) or almond milk (212)
12 ◆ ● ●	*leftover* cinnamon & fennel braised pork, *leftover* roasted butternut squash mash, *leftover* spiced applesauce	[make ahead] curried chicken salad with apples (80), carrot-ginger soup (126)	[make-ahead] slow cooker chicken adobo (70), creamy mushroom soup (132)	*leftover* apple spice "granola," *leftover* coconut or almond milk
13 ■ ● ● ●	southwestern breakfast skillet (52), avocado crema (196)	*leftover* curried chicken salad with apples, *leftover* carrot-ginger soup	bbq chicken (81), green bean casserole (154; *uses leftover* creamy mushroom soup)	hard-boiled egg + salt & vinegar kale chips (172)
14 ● ● ◆	butternut squash pancakes (62), spiced buttery apple spread (203)	*leftover* bbq chicken, *leftover* green bean casserole	smoky grilled pork chops with cookout coleslaw (106), brussels sprouts with crispy capers & bacon (138)	pesto deviled eggs (162) + *leftover* salt & vinegar kale chips

KEY
- ● Eggs
- ● Poultry
- ◆ Pork
- ■ Lamb
- ■ Beef/Bison
- ▲ Seafood

NOTES

*   choose any green vegetable from your Yes foods list on page 40

^   choose any of The 21DSD salad dressings

Add a starchy vegetable if you are following modifications that direct you to do so.

Bold italicized items are optional—you can add them or leave them out.

Icons denote the main protein source in meals for planning purposes. Snacks are optional.

THE 21-DAY SUGAR DETOX COOKBOOK • DIANE SANFILIPPO

level 3

DAY	BREAKFAST	LUNCH	DINNER	SNACK
15 ● ◆ ▲	[make-ahead] nutty cinnamon crumb cake (182), 2 eggs any style or 3oz protein of choice	*leftover* smoky grilled pork chops with cookout coleslaw, *leftover* brussels sprouts with crispy capers & bacon	cilantro shrimp stir-fry (122), garlic & green onion cauli-rice (136)	21DSD-friendly fruit + sunbutter (164) or nut butter
16 ● ◆ ■	*leftover* nutty cinnamon crumb cake, 2 eggs any style or 3oz protein of choice	[make-ahead] portuguese green soup (130)	chorizo burgers with spicy red onions (98), green salad* & dressing^	21DSD-friendly fruit + *leftover* sunbutter / nut butter
17 ● ● ●	mushroom & green onion frittata (58), avocado	*leftover* portuguese green soup	lemon ginger chicken (72), asian sautéed greens (140)	apple spice "granola" (178), coconut (210) or almond milk (212)
18 ● ● ◆	smoothie of choice (49–51) with 2 eggs any style or 3oz protein of choice	*leftover* lemon ginger chicken, *leftover* asian sautéed greens	italian sausage & peppers (104), roasted garlic parsnip mash (148)	*leftover* apple spice "granola," *leftover* coconut or almond milk
19 ● ● ●	smoothie of choice (49–51) with 2 eggs any style or 3oz protein of choice	*leftover* italian sausage & peppers, *leftover* roasted garlic parsnip mash	tandoori chicken skewers (74), moroccan cauli-rice pilaf (137)	turkey jerky (174) + choice of nuts or smoky lime nut mix (171)
20 ● ◆ ● ■	[make-ahead] breakfast sausage & biscuit sandwich (60), steamed green vegetable*	*leftover* tandoori chicken skewers, *leftover* moroccan cauli-rice pilaf	beef larb (thai lettuce wraps) (90)	*leftover* turkey jerky + *leftover* smoky lime nut mix
21 ● ■ ●	2 eggs any style or 3oz protein of choice with steamed green vegetable*	*leftover* beef larb (thai lettuce wraps)	chicken pot pie (66), mixed greens salad* & dressing^	sundried tomato hummus (169), veggies

KEY
- ● Eggs
- ● Poultry
- ◆ Pork
- ■ Lamb
- ■ Beef/Bison
- ▲ Seafood

NOTES

*   choose any green vegetable from your Yes foods list on page 40

^   choose any of The 21DSD salad dressings

Add a starchy vegetable if you are following modifications that direct you to do so.

Bold italicized items are optional—you can add them or leave them out.

Icons denote the main protein source in meals for planning purposes. Snacks are optional.

THE 21 DAY SUGAR DETOX

LEVEL 3

YES FOODS *eat plenty of these foods for 21 days*

MEAT, FISH, & EGGS
including but not limited to:
ALL meats, including deli and cured meats like bacon, pancetta, prosciutto, etc. (see page 226 for the best brands)
ALL seafood
Eggs

VEGETABLES
Artichokes/sunchokes
Asparagus
Broccoli
Brussels sprouts
Cabbage
Carrots
Cauliflower
Celery/celery root
Chard
Collards
Cucumber
Eggplant
Garlic
Ginger
Green beans
Horseradish
Jicama
Kale
Leeks
Lettuce, *all leafy greens*
Mushrooms
Onions
Parsnips
Peppers, *all varieties*
Radicchio
Radishes
Rutabaga
Snow/snap peas
Spaghetti squash
Spinach
Tomato
Turnips
Yellow squash
Zucchini

FRUIT
review the Limit foods for more fruit choices!
Lemon
Lime

NUTS/SEEDS
whole, flour, or butters
Almonds
Brazil nuts
Cocoa/cacao (100%), nibs
Chia seeds
Coconut, *all unsweetened forms are okay—coconut sugar is a NO*
Filberts (hazelnuts)
Flaxseed
Hemp seeds
Macadamia nuts
Pecans
Pistachios
Pumpkin seeds
Sunflower seeds
Sesame seeds, tahini
Walnuts

FATS & OILS
review the guide on page 228
Animal fats
Butter, ghee, clarified butter
Avocados, avocado oil
Coconut oil
Flax oil
Olives, olive oil
Sesame oil

BEVERAGES
Almond milk, unsweetened/homemade (page 212)
Coconut milk, coconut cream, full-fat
Coffee, espresso
Mineral water
Seltzer, club soda
Teas: herbal, green, black, white, etc., unsweetened
Water

CONDIMENTS/MISC.
Broth, homemade only (recipe on page 208)
Coconut aminos
Sweetener-Free Ketchup (recipe on page 216) *no store-bought ketchups are allowed*
Extracts: vanilla, almond, vanilla bean, etc.
Hummus made from cauliflower (recipe on page 169
Healthy Homemade Mayonnaise (recipe on page 219) *do your best to avoid others*
Mustard, gluten-free varieties
Nutritional/Brewer's yeast (Lewis Labs brand)
Salad dressings, homemade
Spices & herbs: all are OK; check premixed blends for hidden ingredients
Vinegars: apple cider, balsamic, distilled, red wine, rice, sherry, white

SUPPLEMENTS
Protein powder, 100% pure with NO other ingredients (e.g., 100% egg white or hemp)
Fermented cod liver oil, with or without flavor (one exception to the no-sweetener rule!)
Pure vitamin or mineral supplements

DON'T SEE THE FOOD YOU WANT TO EAT ON THE LIST?
Review "Is it a Yes food?" on page 19.

MODIFICATIONS
If you are following the Energy or Autoimmune tracks, see the meal plan modifications on pages 42–43 for additional notes.

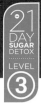

LIMIT FOODS *these are Yes foods with portion size limits*

VEGETABLES & STARCHES
1 cup serving per day is allowed

Acorn squash
Beets
Butternut squash
Green peas
Pumpkin
Winter squash (assorted)

FRUIT
1 piece per day is allowed

Bananas, green-tipped/
   not quite ripe only
Grapefruit
Green/Granny Smith
   apples

BEVERAGES
1 cup total per day is allowed

Coconut juice, coconut
   water (no added sweet-
   eners)
Kombucha, home-
   brewed or store-bought
   (see recommended
   brands on page 226)

NO FOODS *do not eat these foods for 21 days*

REFINED CARBOHYDRATES
Bagels
Bread
Breadsticks
Brownies
Cake
Candy
Cereal/granola
Chips
Cookies
Couscous
Crackers
Croissants
Cupcakes
Muffins
Oats
Orzo
Pasta
Pastries
Pita
Pizza
Popcorn
Rice cakes
Rolls
Tortillas, tortilla chips

VEGETABLES & STARCHES
Cassava
Corn, polenta, grits
Plantains
Soybeans/edamame
Sweet potatoes/yams
Tapioca, whole & flour
Taro

FRUITS
*review the Yes and Limit foods
lists for included fruits*
Fresh & dried

GRAINS/LEGUMES
Amaranth
Arrowroot
Barley
Beans: black, fava,
   garbanzo (chickpeas),
   navy, pinto, red
Buckwheat
Flours made from grains
   or beans (chickpeas,
   lentils, etc.)
Kamut
Lentils
Millet
Quinoa
Rice (brown, white, wild)
Rye
Sorghum
Soybeans/edamame
   (including miso, natto,
   tempeh, tofu, and soy
   sauce)
Spelt
Wheat

NUTS/NUT BUTTERS
Cashew
Peanut

DAIRY
Cheese, cream cheese,
   cottage cheese
Milk
Half & half
Heavy cream
Sour cream
Yogurt/kefir

SWEETENERS OF ANY KIND
None are allowed!

ANYTHING "DIET," SUGAR-FREE, OR ARTIFICIALLY SWEETENED
This means no gum,
either!

SUPPLEMENTS
Anything that includes
   sugar, sweeteners, or
   sugar alcohols (xylitol,
   for example)
Shakeology and other
   similar blends
Supplements that con-
   tain soy, corn, or wheat

BEVERAGES
All alcohol
Coffee "drinks" or shakes,
   presweetened
Juice
Milk, soy/rice/oat
Soda (regular & diet)
Sweet-tasting drinks
   (besides herbal teas)
Protein powders that
   have more than one
   ingredient (see Yes food
   supplements)

CONDIMENTS/MISC.
Broth/stock in a box/can
Hummus made from
   garbanzo beans
Ketchup, store-bought
Mayonnaise, store-bought
Salad dressings, pre-
   made/store-bought
Soy sauce, tamari

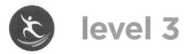
additional notes for those who need more carbohydrates

THESE MODIFICATIONS MAY BE RIGHT FOR YOU IF YOU

- live a very active lifestyle or work at a physically demanding job
- participate in high-intensity physical activity or exercise regularly (for example, interval training, CrossFit-style workouts, endurance athletics, or cardio/aerobic activity at moderate to high intensity for more than 20 minutes at a time; yoga alone doesn't typically require these modifications)
- are pregnant or nursing

With the Energy Modifications, you will need to add to your meal plan starchy carbohydrate vegetables that are considered No foods for those who do not fit the modification requirements listed above.

STARCHY CARBOHYDRATE VEGETABLES
amount varies based on your activity level and energy requirements; see page 230 for a list of these foods
Add 30–50 grams of carbohydrates to a *minimum* of one meal per day, especially after exercise. This means 1/2 to 1 cup of mashed sweet potato or plantain, for example. You should also use the one piece of fruit per day included for all Level 3 detoxers to reach this carbohydrate goal.

If you train very hard (at high intensity or more than once a day), you may need to make this modification for *each instance* of exercise—meaning more than one meal or snack will include up to 30–50 grams of dense carbohydrates.

You may adjust when you eat your extra carbs. For example, if sweet potato is listed at lunch but you generally feel better including your additional carbs at dinner, you can absolutely do that. In general, adding more carbs later in the day or after activity tends to replenish your fuel better. *This is a highly variable element in your meal planning, and tracking your own energy levels is the best way to decide when to consume your extra carbs.*

RECOMMENDED CARBS PER DAY
Moderately active: 75–150 grams
Highly active: 100–200+ grams
Pregnant/nursing: 100+ grams
These are estimates. If you find that you need more carbs to maintain activity, adjust to your needs.

If you are pregnant or nursing, add these carbohydrate sources as you see fit. Do not limit them assuming it will lead to better results. The goal of this program is a healthy body and a healthy baby, and limiting these foods further is absolutely not necessary! If you find that your milk supply is low or you feel more fatigued than usual, increase your intake of carbohydrate-dense foods as outlined here.

MODIFICATIONS **autoimmune** level 3

additional notes for those who have
autoimmune health conditions

THESE MODIFICATIONS MAY BE RIGHT FOR YOU IF YOU

• have been diagnosed with an autoimmune condition or suspect you may have one

With the Autoimmune Modifications, you will be eliminating several foods from your meal plan that are considered Yes foods for those who do not fit the modification requirements listed above. These foods are common allergens and are generally irritating to digestion. By improving digestive function, immune function can also be improved. If you have an autoimmune condition and have never eliminated these foods, I highly recommend doing so for the 21 days of this program to see how you feel without them, then reintroduce them and track any changes.

EGGS
omit from your meals and snacks
See page 224 for ideas on how to replace eggs in recipes.

NUTS & SEEDS
omit from your meals and snacks
This includes whole nuts, nut butters, seeds, and seed butters. Nuts are highlighted in recipes where they are included, and omissions or substitutions are noted if the recipe can bear the change.

NIGHTSHADE VEGETABLES & SPICES
omit from your meals and snacks
This includes tomatoes, potatoes, peppers (including spices such as paprika, chili powder, and cayenne pepper), and eggplant. Nightshades are highlighted in recipes where they are included, and omissions or substitutions are noted if the recipe can bear the change.

easy **recipes**

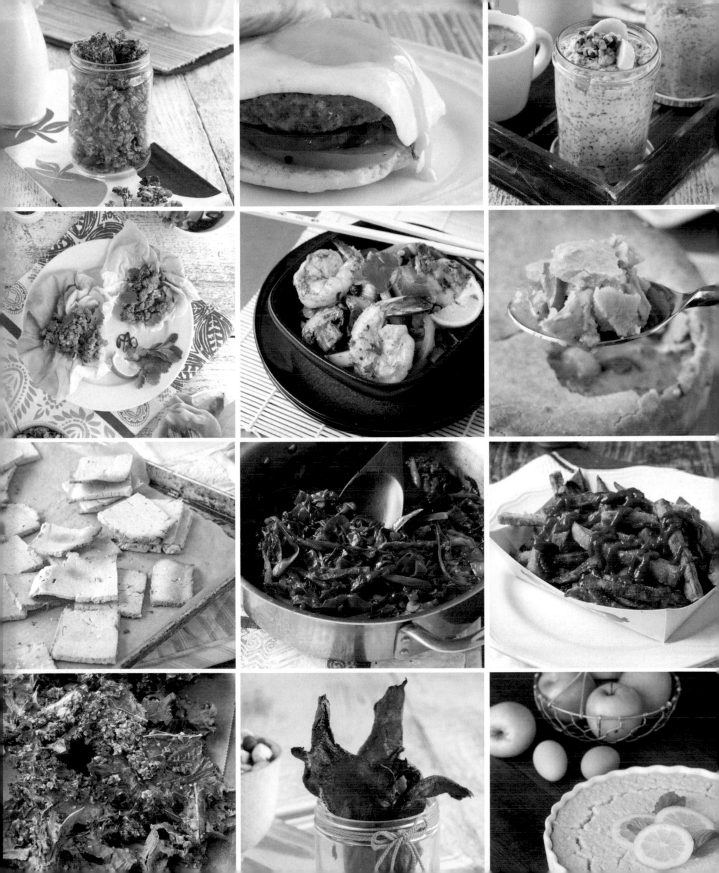

banana vanilla bean n'oatmeal

PREP TIME **15 MINS** • COOK TIME **15 MINS (+3 HRS TO CHILL)** • SERVINGS **4**

NUTS

EGGS

NIGHTSHADES

FODMAPS

SEAFOOD

2 eggs

1 vanilla bean pod

14.5 ounces coconut milk (about 1 3/4 cups), canned* or homemade (page 210)

1/2 cup water

1 green-tipped banana, sliced

1 teaspoon ground cinnamon

pinch of sea salt

1/4 cup chia seeds

chopped nuts (optional, omit for nut-free), banana slices, or more coconut milk, for garnish

Whisk the eggs in a small bowl and set the bowl next to your stove. Slice the vanilla bean pod in half lengthwise, then, using the tip of a paring knife, scrape out the seeds. Put the scraped-out seeds, bean pod, coconut milk, and water in a saucepan and heat slowly over medium heat, stirring often. Once the mixture begins to simmer, stir more frequently; continue to simmer for 5 minutes. Remove the vanilla bean pod and discard. Slowly pour a ladleful of the hot coconut milk mixture into the eggs as you whisk rapidly to incorporate. Then pour the coconut milk egg mixture back into the saucepan while continuing to whisk. Cook for 5 to 10 minutes, stirring occasionally, or until a spoon remains coated when dipped into the mixture.

Pour the entire mixture into a blender, add the banana, and blend until smooth, approximately 1 to 2 minutes. Add the cinnamon, salt, and chia seeds and pulse a few times or until evenly dispersed.

Divide the mixture into 4 serving bowls, jars, or glasses; cover; and refrigerate for at least 3 hours, preferably overnight. Garnish with chopped nuts, banana slices, or more coconut milk poured over the top. To serve warm, reheat in a saucepan over low heat until warmed through.

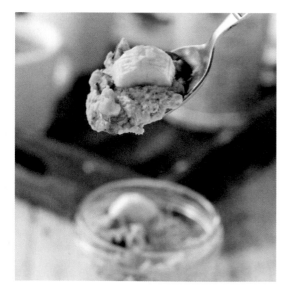

INGREDIENT TIP

*Check out pages 226-227 for a list of recommended brands.

EGG-FREE?

Omit the eggs. Blend all the ingredients in a blender, adding the chia seeds at the very end. Pour into containers and refrigerate for at least 4 hours. The consistency will be more like yogurt. ●

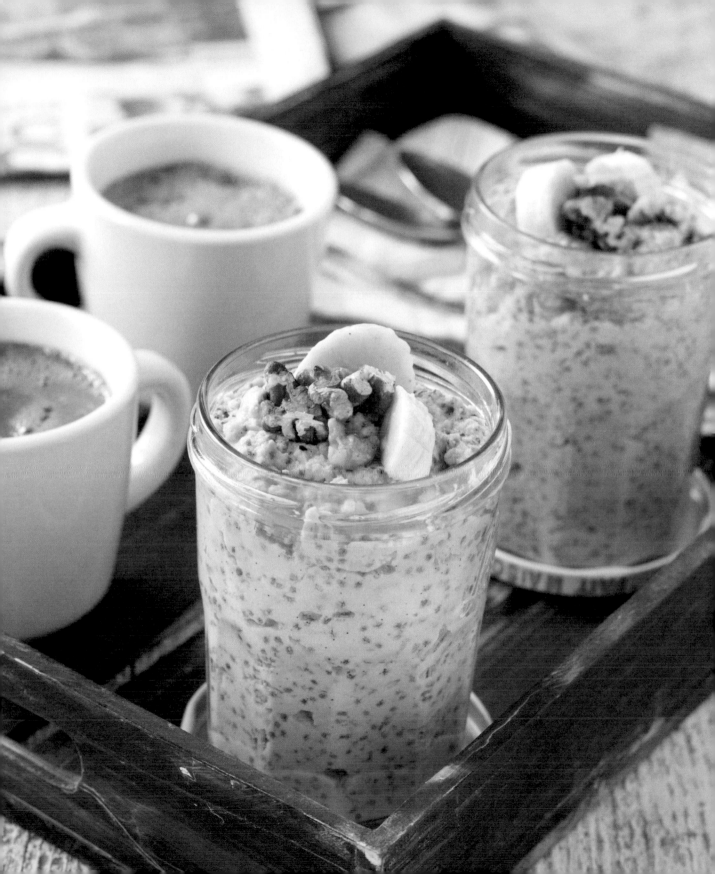

NUTS

EGGS

NIGHTSHADES

FODMAPS

SEAFOOD

carrot-apple skillet breakfast hash

PREP TIME **15 MINS** • COOK TIME **25 TO 30 MINS** • SERVINGS **4**

4 slices bacon, chopped

4 carrots, peeled (2 cups shredded)

1 green apple, peeled (1 cup shredded)

1 pound ground chicken, turkey, or pork

1 to 2 tablespoons Italian Sausage Spice Blend (page 222)

sea salt and black pepper to taste

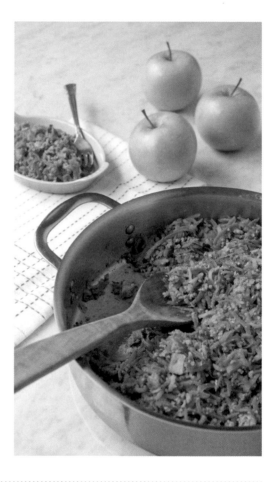

In a large sauté pan or skillet over medium heat, cook the bacon for 8 to 10 minutes, stirring occasionally, until the fat has rendered off and the meat becomes crispy. While the bacon cooks, shred the carrots and green apple.

Once the bacon has cooked, add the chicken to the pan and season with 1 tablespoon of the Spice Blend, breaking up the meat with a heat-safe spatula or wooden spoon. Allow it to cook, stirring occasionally, for about 8 minutes or until the meat is cooked through (there should be no pink remaining). Taste and add more Spice Blend and salt and pepper if desired.

Reduce the heat to medium-low and add the carrots and apple to the pan. Stir to combine, cover, and cook until the carrots are tender, about 5 minutes. Remove the lid and allow any liquid to evaporate out of the pan before serving.

Use shredded sweet potatoes instead of carrots.

apple ginger green smoothie

PREP TIME **5 MINS** • SERVINGS **2**

2 cups packed spinach

2 cups full-fat coconut milk, canned* or homemade (page 210), or Almond Milk (page 212)

1 cup ice

1/2 avocado

juice of 1 lemon

1 (1/2-inch to 1-inch) piece of fresh ginger, peeled and minced

1 green apple, peeled, cored, and chopped

1/2 to 1 cup water

NUTS

EGGS

NIGHTSHADES

FODMAPS

SEAFOOD

INGREDIENT TIP
*Check out pages 226–227 for a list of recommended brands.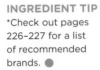

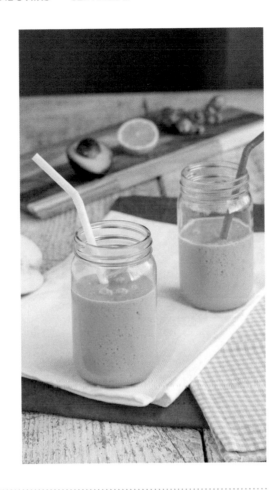

Place all the ingredients in a blender, adding the water as needed to reach the desired consistency. Blend until smooth, about 60 seconds.

apple pie smoothie

PREP TIME **5 MINS** • SERVINGS **1 TO 2**

1 cup full-fat coconut milk, canned* or homemade (page 210)

1/2 cup water

1 green apple, peeled, cored, and chopped

2 tablespoons almond butter*

1 teaspoon pure vanilla extract

1 1/2 teaspoons ground cinnamon

2 dashes nutmeg, for garnish

small handful of ice (optional)

1 to 2 scoops 100% grass-fed whey protein powder or other 100% single-ingredient protein powder** (optional)

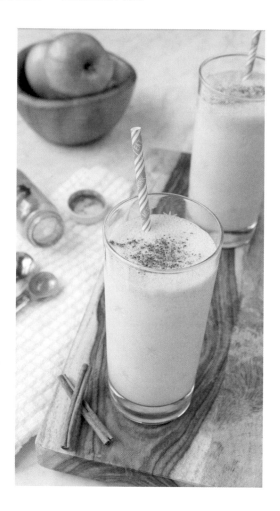

INGREDIENT TIPS
*Check out pages 226–227 for a list of recommended brands.

**Review your Yes/No Foods List for details on protein powder.

NUT FREE?
Use Sunbutter (page 164) or coconut butter instead of almond butter. ●

Purée all the ingredients in a blender until smooth.

 Use coconut butter instead of almond butter.

pumpkin spice smoothie

PREP TIME **5 MINS** • SERVINGS **1 TO 2**

1 cup full-fat coconut milk, canned* or homemade (page 210)

1/2 cup water

1 green-tipped banana, frozen

1/4 cup canned pumpkin

1 teaspoon pure vanilla extract

1 teaspoon ground cinnamon

1 teaspoon pumpkin pie spice

small handful of ice (optional)

1 to 2 scoops 100% grass-fed whey protein powder or other 100% single-ingredient protein powder** (optional)

NUTS

EGGS

NIGHTSHADES

FODMAPS

SEAFOOD

INGREDIENT TIPS

*Check out pages 226–227 for a list of recommended brands.

**Review your Yes/No Foods List for details on protein powder. ●

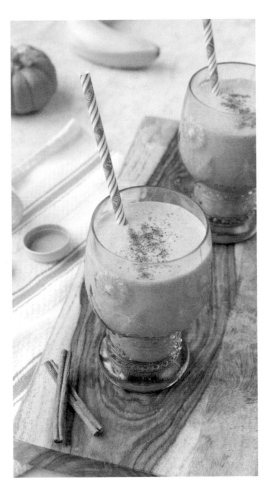

Purée all the ingredients in a blender until smooth.

Replace the pumpkin with sweet potato.

southwestern breakfast skillet

PREP TIME **15 MINS** • COOK TIME **25 MINS** • SERVINGS **4**

NUTS

EGGS

NIGHTSHADES

FODMAPS

SEAFOOD

1 tablespoon coconut oil or other cooking fat*

1/2 cup diced red onion

1/2 cup diced yellow bell pepper

1/2 cup diced red bell pepper

1 jalapeño pepper, minced (optional)

1 pound ground beef, bison, turkey, or chicken

2 tablespoons Southwestern Spice Blend (page 223), divided

4 large parsnips, shredded (4 cups)

1 (4-ounce) can diced green chilies

6 eggs

sea salt and black pepper to taste

2 tablespoons or more Avocado Crema (page 196)

1/4 cup chopped cilantro

In a large oven-safe skillet over medium-high heat, melt the coconut oil and cook the onion, bell peppers, and jalapeño for 1 minute. Crumble in the ground meat and sprinkle with 1 tablespoon of the Spice Blend. Stir to combine and cook until the meat is browned and mostly cooked through, about 10 minutes.

Add the shredded parsnips and can of green chilies, sprinkle with the remaining 1 tablespoon of the Spice Blend, and stir to combine. Continue cooking until the parsnips start to soften (don't allow them to get too soft), about 3 to 5 minutes.

Place the oven rack in the top position and preheat the broiler to low.

Make 6 wells in the meat-parsnip mixture and crack an egg into each one. Put the pan under the broiler and cook for about 5 minutes or until the whites are cooked through and the yolks are cooked to the desired doneness.

Add salt and pepper to taste and garnish with Avocado Crema and cilantro.

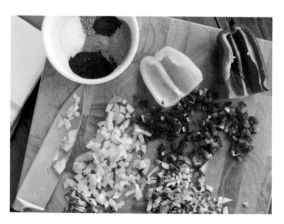

INGREDIENT TIP
*Refer to page 228 to see which fats are best for cooking. ●

 Use shredded sweet potatoes instead of parsnips.

 Omit the ground beef.

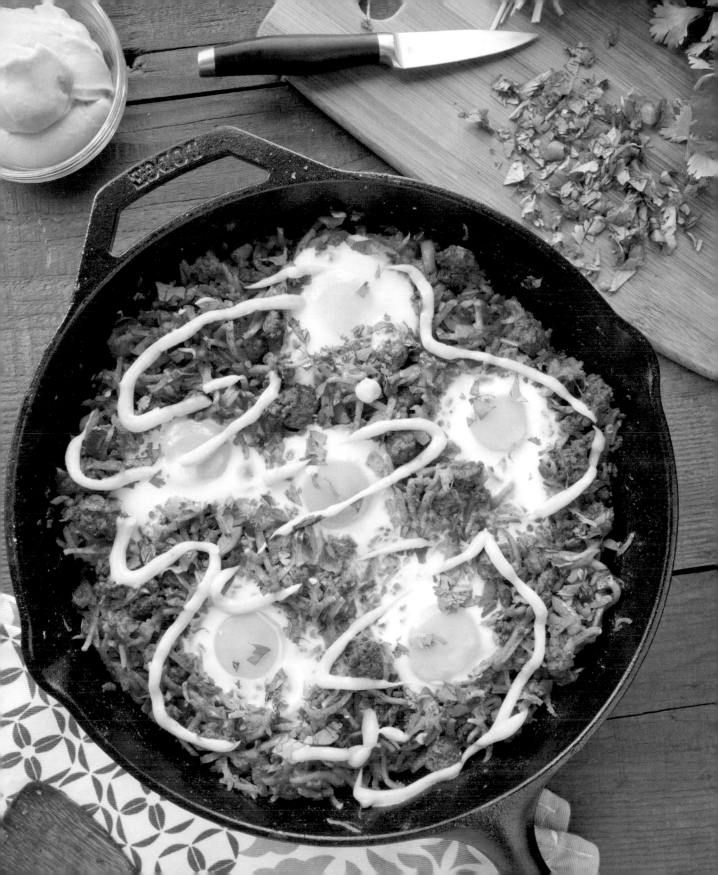

worth-the-wait crustless quiche

PREP TIME **10 MINS** • COOK TIME **45 MINS (+ 45 MINS FOR CARAMELIZED ONIONS)** • SERVINGS **4**

NUTS

EGGS

NIGHTSHADES

FODMAPS

SEAFOOD

Caramelized Onions
(page 200)

1 tablespoon cooking fat,*
for greasing the baking
dish

8 slices bacon, chopped

8 eggs

sea salt and black pepper

Prepare the Caramelized Onions, if you haven't
already.

Preheat the oven to 350°F. Grease a 9-by-11-
inch casserole dish.

In a large skillet over medium heat, cook the
bacon for 8 to 10 minutes until the fat has
rendered off and the meat becomes crispy.
Using a slotted spoon, place the bacon on a
paper towel to drain, leaving the fat in the pan.

In a mixing bowl, whisk the eggs and season
with salt and pepper. Mix the bacon into the
beaten eggs, then add the Caramelized Onions.
Pour the egg mixture into the prepared
casserole dish and bake for 30 to 40 minutes or
until the eggs puff up and the edges become
brown and pull away from the sides of the pan.

This quiche freezes and reheats well in a
toaster oven once defrosted overnight.

Serve with a mixed greens salad or sautéed
greens.

INGREDIENT TIP
*Refer to page 228 to see which fats are best
for cooking.

CHEF NOTE
Caramelized onions are very easy to make,
but they take a long time! I highly recommend
making a double batch to keep on hand for
recipes like this one and the BBQ Sauce on
page 199. ●

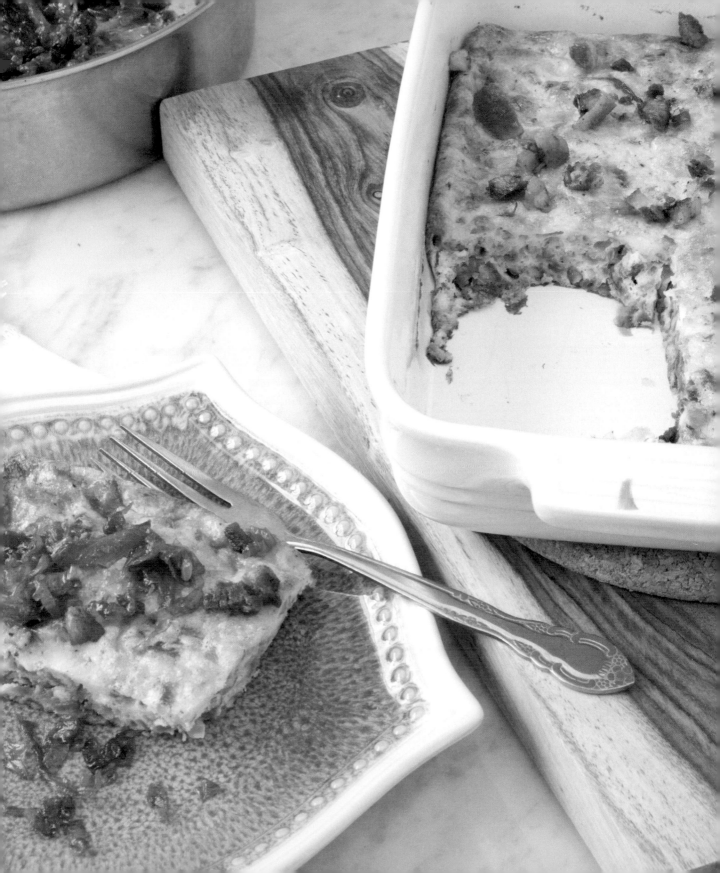

MAIN
DISHES

NUTS
EGGS
NIGHTSHADES
FODMAPS
SEAFOOD

pizza frittata

PREP TIME **15 MINS** • COOK TIME **35 MINS** • SERVINGS **6**

1/2 pound ground pork

1 tablespoon Italian Sausage Spice Blend (page 222)

8 eggs

1 1/4 teaspoons sea salt, divided

1/2 teaspoon black pepper

1/2 cup tomato sauce

1/2 teaspoon dried basil

1/2 teaspoon dried oregano

1/2 teaspoon granulated garlic

1 tablespoon cooking fat*

1 bell pepper, sliced

5 mushrooms, sliced

3 green onions (scallions), sliced

1/2 cup sliced olives

INGREDIENT TIP
*Refer to page 228 to see which fats are best for cooking. ●

Preheat the oven to 400°F.

Heat a large oven-safe skillet over medium heat. While the skillet is heating up, combine the ground pork and Spice Blend in a mixing bowl and mix them together until the spices are evenly distributed. Add the meat to the skillet and cook until just a little pink is visible, about 10 minutes, breaking up the meat with a heat-safe spatula or wooden spoon as it cooks. Remove the pork from the pan and set aside. (Do not wash the pan; you will use it again.)

In a small bowl, whisk together the eggs, 1 teaspoon of the salt, and the pepper. In another small bowl, stir together the tomato sauce, basil, oregano, granulated garlic, and the remaining 1/4 teaspoon of salt. Set both bowls aside.

Melt the cooking fat in the pan (the same pan you used to cook the pork) over medium heat, then add the bell pepper and cook until it starts to soften, about 5 minutes. Add the mushrooms and cook for 2 minutes or until they soften slightly. Put the meat back into the pan along with the majority of the green onions (reserving some for garnish) and the olives and stir to combine all the ingredients.

Pour in the egg mixture and tilt the pan back and forth until the eggs cover the entire bottom of the pan. If necessary, give the ingredients a gentle stir to distribute them evenly. Let cook for about 5 minutes or until the edges begin to set.

Drizzle the tomato sauce mixture over the eggs, then place the pan in the oven and cook for 8 to 10 minutes or until the eggs are set. To check, use a knife to make a cut in the center of the frittata—if raw egg runs along the cut, cook for another 2 to 3 minutes and check again.

Let sit for 5 minutes before slicing and serving.

 Omit the pork, stir cooked spinach into the egg mixture before adding it to the skillet.

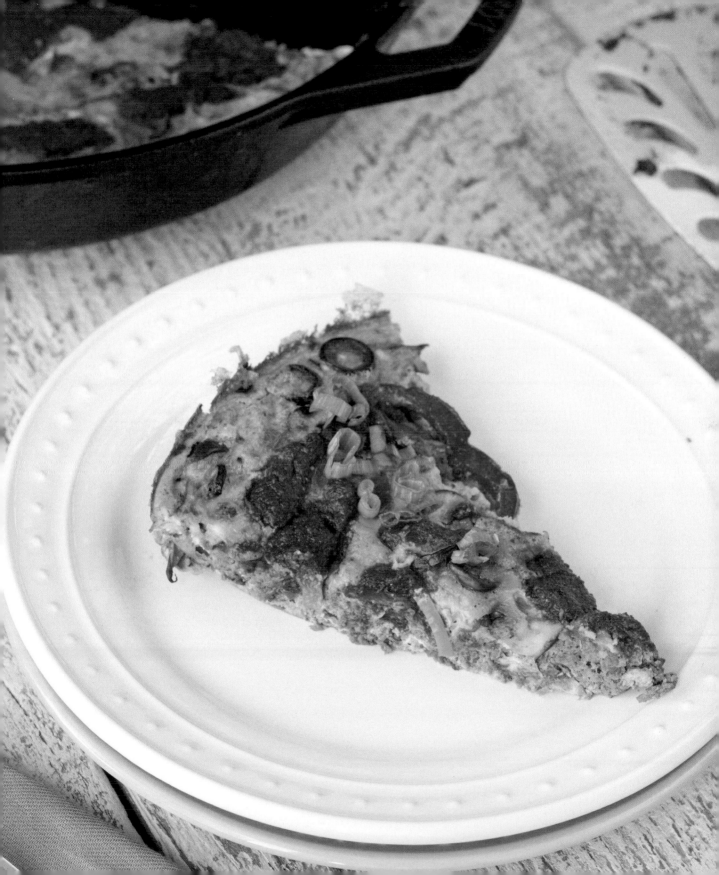

mushroom & green onion frittata

PREP TIME 10 MINS • COOK TIME 30 MINS • SERVINGS 4

NUTS

EGGS

NIGHTSHADES

FODMAPS

SEAFOOD

8 cremini mushrooms

1 tablespoon bacon fat, ghee, or coconut oil

sea salt and black pepper

4 green onions (scallions), sliced into 1/4-inch pieces

1/2 teaspoon dried thyme (optional)

8 eggs

2 tablespoons full-fat coconut milk, canned* or homemade (page 210), or Almond Milk (page 212)

Sweetener-Free Ketchup (page 216, optional, omit for nightshade free), for serving

Preheat the oven to 350°F.

Slice the mushrooms into thin strips. In a large cast-iron or other oven-safe skillet, melt the cooking fat over medium heat. Cook the mushrooms in the fat for about 10 minutes, stirring occasionally, until they have browned and released their moisture; season with a dash of salt and pepper a few minutes into the cooking process. Add the green onions and dried thyme to the pan and cook for an additional minute.

In a mixing bowl, whisk the eggs with the milk and season liberally with salt and pepper. Pour the eggs into the skillet with the vegetables and cook for 2 minutes over medium heat, then place the skillet in the oven. Bake for 15 to 20 minutes or until the eggs puff up and the edges become brown and pull away from the sides of the pan.

Serve topped with Sweetener-Free Ketchup, page 216.

INGREDIENT TIP

*Check out pages 226–227 for a list of recommended brands. ●

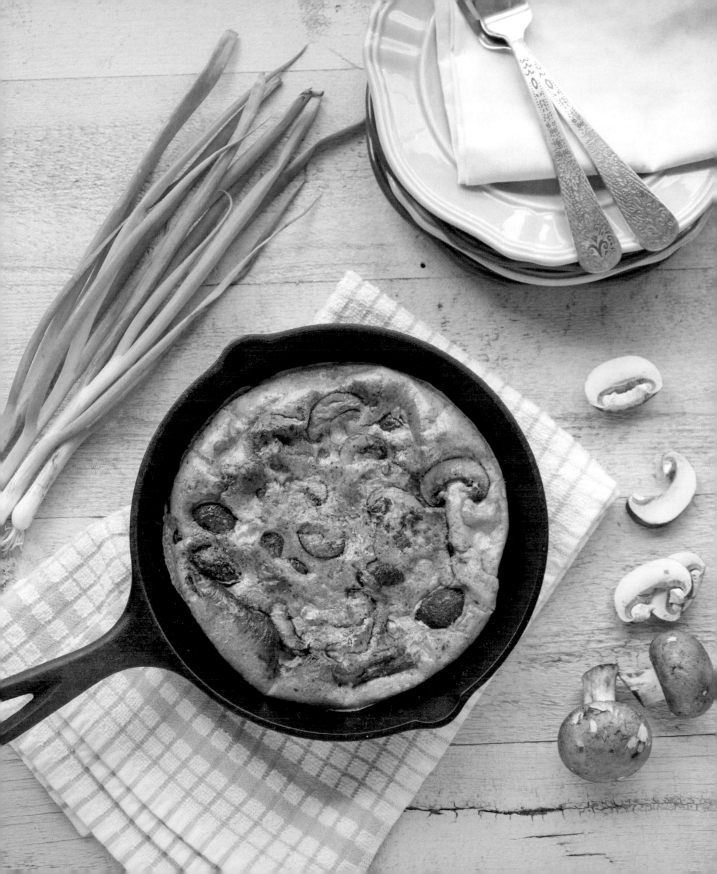

breakfast sausage
& biscuit sandwich

PREP TIME **10 MINS** • COOK TIME **15 TO 18 MINS** • SERVINGS **4**

NUTS

EGGS

NIGHTSHADES

FODMAPS

SEAFOOD

FOR THE SAUSAGE

1 pound ground pork or
   other meat

2 tablespoons Breakfast
   Sausage Spice Blend
   (page 223)

1 to 2 tablespoons cooking
   fat, as needed

2 bell peppers, sliced

sea salt and black pepper

4 eggs

1 recipe "Buttermilk" Buns
   (page 166)

In a mixing bowl, combine the meat and Spice
Blend evenly with your hands, taking care not
to overmix it or the meat will become tough.
Form the meat into 4 patties and cook in a
large skillet over medium heat for 4 minutes
per side or until cooked through. Remove
the patties from the skillet, leaving any fat
remaining in the pan. Add additional fat if
needed (you should have about 1 tablespoon of
fat in the pan).

Add the bell peppers to the pan and season
with salt and pepper. Sauté the peppers until
they become soft and slightly browned on the
edges, about 5 minutes.

Either in a separate skillet or in the same pan
after the peppers are finished cooking, cook the
eggs to your liking over medium heat, adding
cooking fat to the pan as needed to prevent
sticking. (The eggs will take 3 to 5 minutes to
cook, depending on how you prepare them.)

Assemble a sandwich by placing one bun
on the plate, then layering the peppers and a
sausage patty, and finally topping it off with an
egg. Repeat with the remaining buns, peppers,
patties, and eggs.

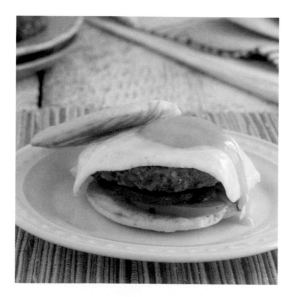

NIGHTSHADE FREE?

Use the Italian Sausage Spice Blend (page
222) instead of the Breakfast Sausage Spice
Blend and omit the bell peppers.

CHEF NOTE

To make this recipe fast and easy for your
morning meal, cook the sausage, peppers,
and buns ahead of time and cook the eggs
to order in the morning while reheating the
rest of the ingredients in a 300°F oven for 10
minutes. ●

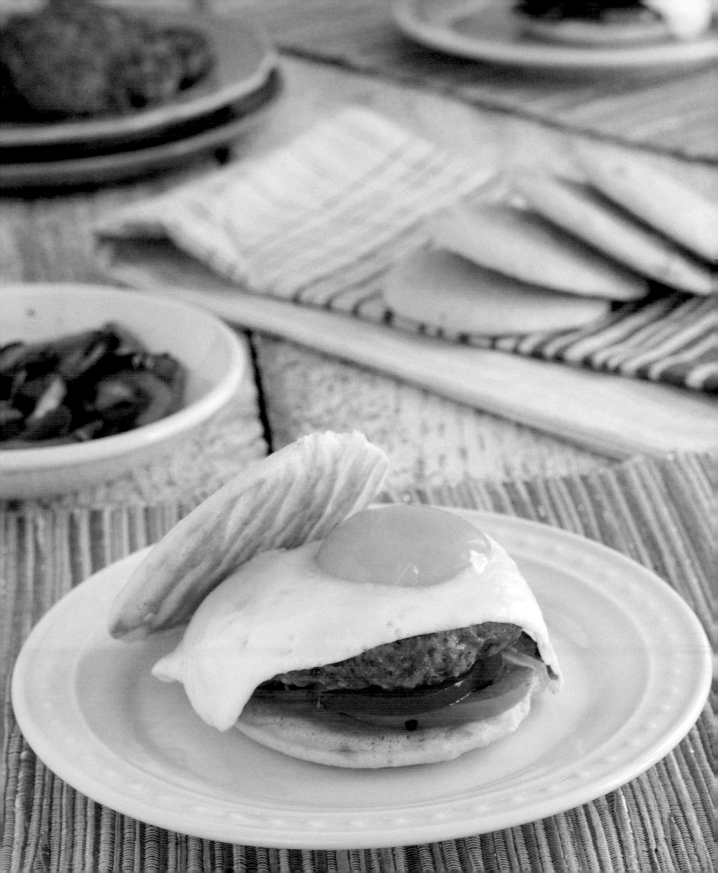

butternut squash pancakes

PREP TIME **10 MINS** • COOK TIME **15 MINS (+ 20 MINS TO COOK SQUASH)** • SERVINGS **4**

• YIELD **16 4-INCH PANCAKES**

NUTS

EGGS

NIGHTSHADES

FODMAPS

SEAFOOD

1 cup steamed and mashed butternut squash

4 eggs

2 cups almond flour*

1 cup full-fat coconut milk, canned* or homemade (page 210)

4 teaspoons ground cinnamon

1 teaspoon ground nutmeg

1/2 teaspoon ground cloves

1/2 teaspoon ground ginger

2 tablespoons coconut flour*

4 teaspoons pure vanilla extract

1 tablespoon coconut oil

Spiced Buttery Apple Spread (page 203), for serving

In a food processor or large blender, combine all the ingredients except the coconut oil and Spiced Buttery Apple Spread and blend until smooth.

In a large skillet, heat the coconut oil over medium heat until hot. Drop about 1/4 cup of batter at a time into 4-inch circles (the batter should yield about 16 pancakes total). Cook for 1 1/2 to 2 minutes on the first side, or until the top side starts to firm up. Most of the cooking is done on this side to help the pancakes flip more easily. Quickly slide a spatula under each pancake and flip. Cook for an additional minute or until cooked through.

Serve with Spiced Buttery Apple Spread.

INGREDIENT TIP
*Check out pages 226-227 for a list of recommended brands.

CHEF NOTE
This batter tends to be quite thick, so you will need to use a spoon to spread the pancakes to size once you drop the batter into the pan. ●

Use cooked sweet potatoes or mashed plantains instead of the butternut squash.

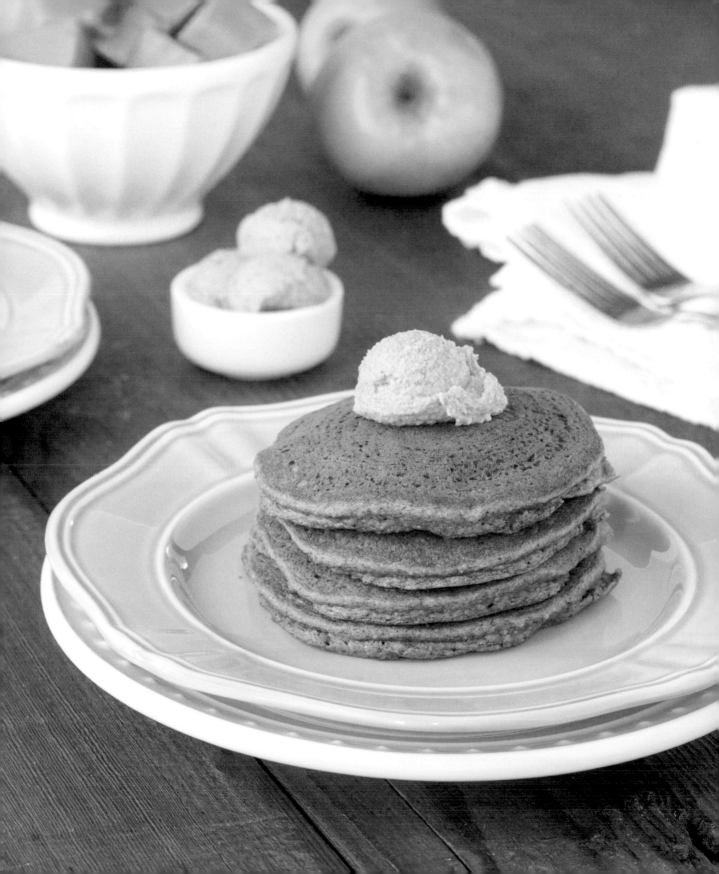

pollo asado

PREP TIME **10 MINS (+ 1 OR MORE HRS TO MARINATE)** • COOK TIME **30 TO 35 MINS** • SERVINGS **4 TO 6**

NUTS

EGGS

NIGHTSHADES

FODMAPS

SEAFOOD

1 yellow onion, sliced

2 shallots, sliced

2 cloves garlic, minced or grated

juice of 4 limes

1/4 cup extra-virgin olive oil

1 tablespoon chili powder

1/4 teaspoon sea salt

1/2 teaspoon black pepper

1 1/2 to 2 pounds boneless, skinless chicken thighs

Basic Cilantro Cauli-Rice (below), for serving

1 lime, cut into wedges, for garnish

1/4 cup chopped fresh cilantro, for garnish

Combine all the ingredients except the chicken, Cauli-Rice, and garnishes in a large mixing bowl and toss to combine. Marinate the chicken in a shallow, nonreactive container for at least an hour.

Preheat the oven to 375°F.

Place the chicken in an oven-safe baking dish and bake for 30 to 35 minutes or until it's white all the way through and reaches an internal temperature of 165°F.

Use two forks to shred the chicken. Serve over Basic Cilantro Cauli-Rice. Garnish with lime wedges and fresh cilantro.

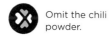

NIGHTSHADE FREE?
Omit the chili powder. ●

 Omit the chili powder.

basic cilantro cauli-rice

PREP TIME **15 MINS** • COOK TIME **5 MINS** • SERVINGS **4 TO 6**

NUTS

EGGS

NIGHTSHADES

FODMAPS

SEAFOOD

1 head cauliflower

1 tablespoon coconut oil or bacon fat

sea salt and black pepper to taste

1/4 cup finely chopped fresh cilantro

OPTIONAL ADD-INS FOR COLOR & VARIETY
as pictured

1/4 cup minced red onion

1/4 cup minced yellow bell pepper (omit for nightshade free)

1 tablespoon coconut oil or bacon fat

Remove the outer leaves and stem from the cauliflower and chop it into large chunks. Shred the cauliflower using a box grater or food processor.

If adding red onion and/or yellow bell pepper, sauté the onion and pepper in 1 tablespoon of coconut oil or bacon fat in a small skillet over medium heat for about 5 minutes or until they become soft and have golden brown edges.

In a large skillet over medium heat, melt the coconut oil or bacon fat, then place the shredded cauliflower in the skillet. Add salt and pepper to taste. Sauté for about 5 minutes or until the cauliflower begins to become translucent, stirring gently to ensure that it cooks through.

Stir in the optional add-ins, place the cooked cauliflower in a serving bowl, and toss with the chopped cilantro before serving.

Make this without the bell pepper add-ins.

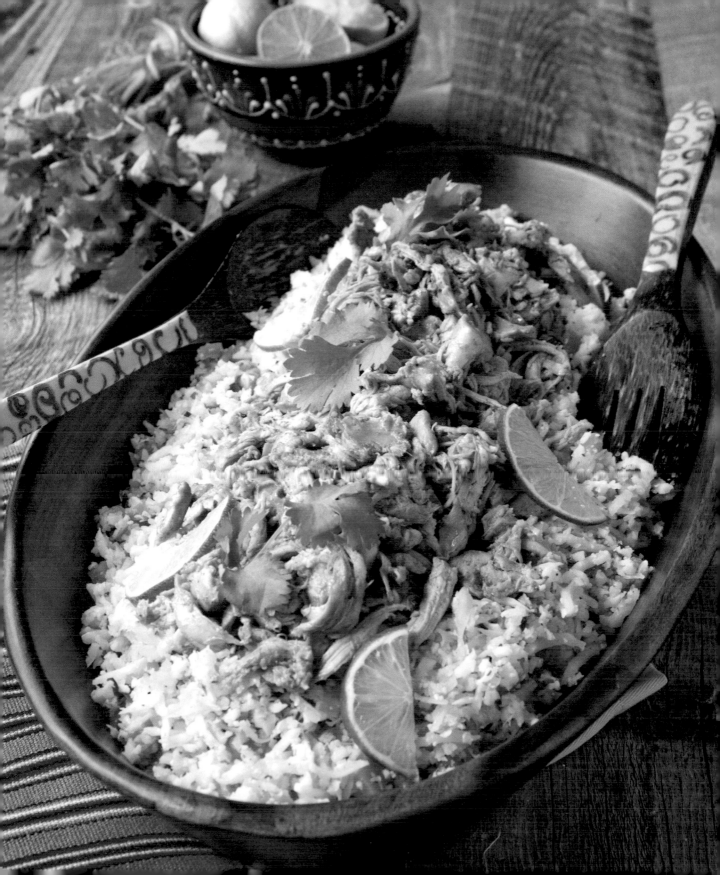

NUTS

EGGS

NIGHTSHADES

FODMAPS

SEAFOOD

chicken pot pie

PREP TIME **30 MINS** • COOK TIME **50 MINS** • SERVINGS **4**

INGREDIENT TIP

*Check out pages 226-227 for a list of recommended brands.

CHEF NOTE

If you don't have any leftover chicken handy, simply bake 1 pound of boneless, skinless chicken with sea salt and black pepper in a 350°F oven for 30-40 minutes until it reaches an internal temperature of 165°F. You can also use a clean-ingredient store-bought rotisserie chicken. ●

CRUST

1 1/3 cups almond flour*

1/2 cup coconut flour*

1/2 teaspoon sea salt

2 eggs, whisked

10 tablespoons butter, lard, or coconut oil frozen

FILLING

8 tablespoons butter or ghee

2 medium carrots, diced (1 cup)

1 medium onion, diced (1 cup)

1 cup chopped fresh green beans (3/4-inch pieces)

2 celery stalks, diced (1 cup)

6 cremini mushroom tops, diced (1 1/2 cups)

1 teaspoon sea salt, plus more if needed

1/2 teaspoon black pepper, plus more if needed

1/2 cup arrowroot flour

14.5 ounces full-fat coconut milk (about 1 3/4 cups), canned* or homemade (page 210)

3 cups Bone Broth, chicken (page 208), warm

1 tablespoon dried parsley

1 teaspoon dried thyme

3 cups shredded cooked chicken (see Chef Note)

1 egg white

2 teaspoons water

Preheat the oven to 400°F.

Make the crust: Combine the almond flour, coconut flour, and salt in a food processor and pulse 4 to 5 times or until combined. Add the eggs and blend until smooth, about 15 to 20 seconds. Take the butter from the freezer and shred using a cheese grater. Add half of the grated butter to the processor and process for 10 seconds. Add the other half of the butter and pulse a few times to just barely combine (small pieces of butter will still be visible). Remove the mixture from the food processor and divide into 4 equal pieces. Press each piece into a ball and wrap individually with plastic wrap. Place the dough balls in the refrigerator to chill.

Make the filling: Melt the butter in a large pot over medium heat. Add the carrots, onion, and green beans and cook for 5 minutes or until the onion becomes translucent. Add the celery and mushrooms and cook until the mushrooms soften, about 3 to 5 minutes.

In a small bowl, mix together the salt, pepper, and arrowroot flour and then sprinkle over the vegetable mixture. Stir until the arrowroot flour is mixed in well—about 2 minutes. Pour in the coconut milk and Bone Broth and bring to a boil, then reduce the heat to medium and simmer until the mixture thickens to the consistency of gravy, about 10 minutes. Add the parsley, thyme, and shredded chicken and simmer for an additional 5 to 10 minutes. Season to taste with more salt and pepper, if needed.

Assemble and bake the pies: Spoon the filling into 4 small soufflé dishes or other individual-sized ovenproof dishes about 12 ounces in capacity, filling them all the way to the top.

Replace the cooked chicken with cooked crab meat.

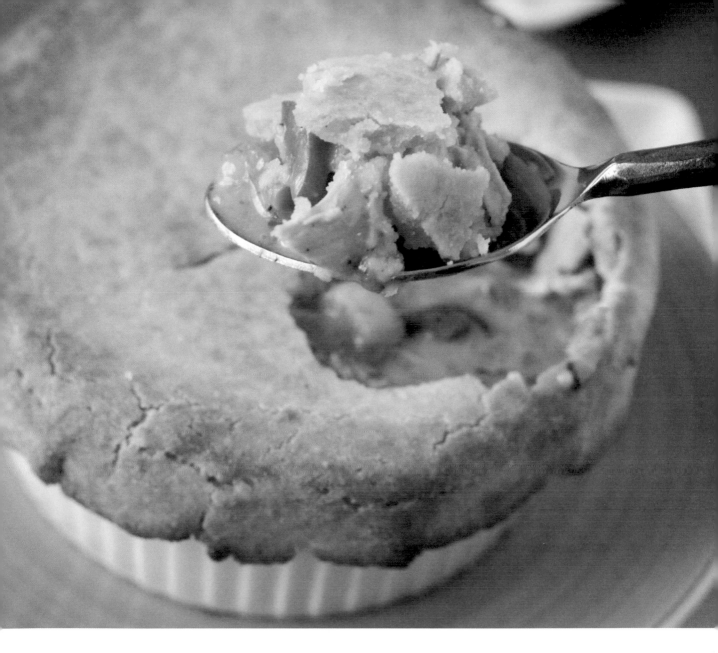

Remove the pie dough from the refrigerator and roll each ball between two pieces of parchment paper until it is just wider than the top of your baking dish (about 1/4-inch thick). Gently place a piece of rolled dough on top of the each baking dish and press down the sides. If any areas crack, press them back together firmly.

Whisk the egg white and water in a small bowl. Use a brush to thinly coat each entire crust with the egg white mixture. Cut slits in the tops of the crusts to let steam escape.

Place the pot pies in the oven on a rimmed sheet pan and bake for 15 to 20 minutes or until the tops are golden brown. Remove from the oven and let cool for 10 to 15 minutes before serving.

artichoke & lemon chicken with capers

PREP TIME **10 MINS** • COOK TIME **20 MINS** • SERVINGS **4**

NUTS

EGGS

NIGHTSHADES

FODMAPS

SEAFOOD

3 lemons

4 tablespoons ghee or coconut oil, divided

2 shallots, sliced

2 cups frozen or canned artichoke hearts, thawed and/or rinsed and drained

1/4 cup capers, drained

2 pounds boneless, skinless chicken thighs

sea salt and black pepper

Juice 2 of the lemons; thinly slice the third lemon into rounds or half moons.

In a large stainless-steel or enameled cast-iron skillet over medium heat, melt 2 tablespoons of the ghee, then add the shallots and sauté them until they are translucent, about 3 to 5 minutes. Add the artichoke hearts, capers, and lemon juice and stir to combine. Move the vegetables to the edges of the skillet and melt the remaining 2 tablespoons of ghee in the center of the skillet.

Season both sides of the chicken thighs liberally with salt and pepper and place them in the center of the pan. Cook for 3 to 4 minutes or until it becomes white around the edges, then flip it to continue cooking the other side.

Reduce the heat to medium-low, move the vegetables over the top of chicken, and place the remaining lemon slices in the pan; continue to cook the chicken until it's white all the way through or reaches an internal temperature of 165°F, about 5 to 8 minutes.

FODMAP-FREE?
Omit the shallots and replace the artichoke hearts with thinly sliced carrots or parsnips.

CHANGE IT UP
You can make this recipe with any parts of the chicken you like; just be sure to cook it to temperature. If using bone-in parts, you may want to cook them skin-side down for a few minutes first, then place the entire skillet (oven-safe only) into a 375°F oven to finish cooking the chicken all the way through. ●

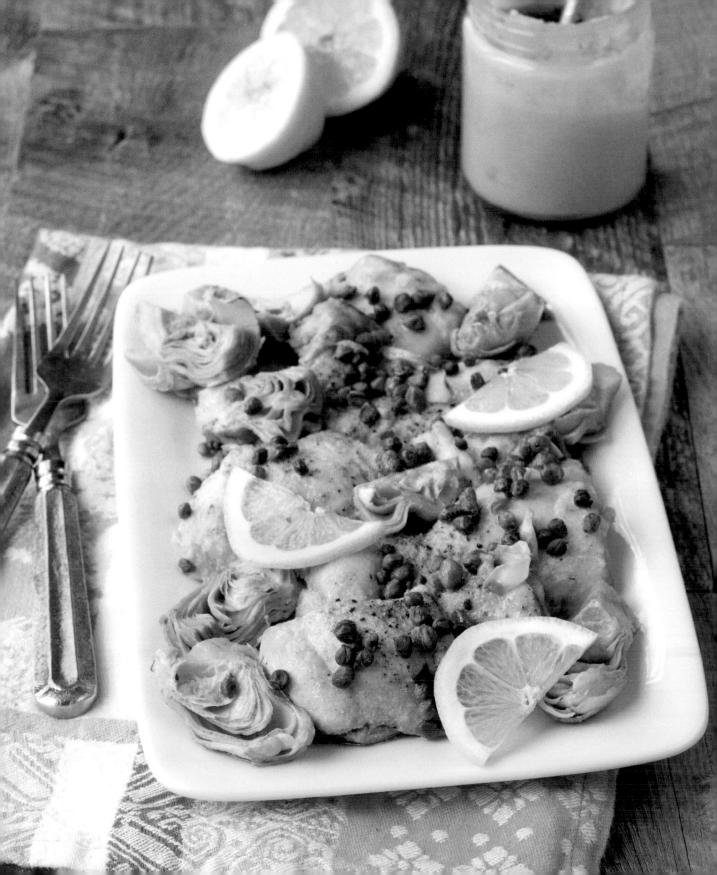

NUTS

EGGS

NIGHTSHADES

FODMAPS

SEAFOOD

slow cooker chicken adobo

PREP TIME **25 MINS** • COOK TIME **4 TO 6 HRS** • SERVINGS **4**

1 large yellow onion, sliced

1 (2-inch) piece of fresh ginger, peeled and thinly sliced

1 head garlic (about 12 cloves), peeled and thinly sliced

2 bay leaves

14.5 ounces full-fat coconut milk (about 1 3/4 cups), canned* or homemade (page 210)

1/2 cup coconut aminos*

1/3 cup apple cider vinegar*

2 teaspoons black pepper, plus more for the chicken

2 tablespoons cooking fat**

3 pounds bone-in chicken thighs

sea salt

Garlic & Green Onion Cauli-Rice, for serving (page 136)

Layer the onion, ginger, garlic, and bay leaves in the bottom of a slow cooker. In a bowl, mix together the coconut milk, coconut aminos, apple cider vinegar, and pepper.

Heat the cooking fat in a skillet over high heat. Season the skin side of the chicken thighs generously with salt and pepper and place them skin side down in the skillet. Cook for about 5 minutes or until the skin is browned.

Transfer the chicken thighs, skin side up, to the slow cooker and pour the coconut milk mixture over the top.

Cook on high for 4 hours or on low for 6 hours.

For a thicker sauce, remove the cooked chicken from the slow cooker, bring the remaining sauce to a boil in a saucepan over medium-high heat, and cook for 20 to 25 minutes to reduce or until desired thickness is achieved.

Serve over Garlic & Green Onion Cauli-Rice.

INGREDIENT TIP
*Check out pages 226–227 for a list of recommended brands.

COOKING TIP
**See page 228 for recommended cooking fats. ●

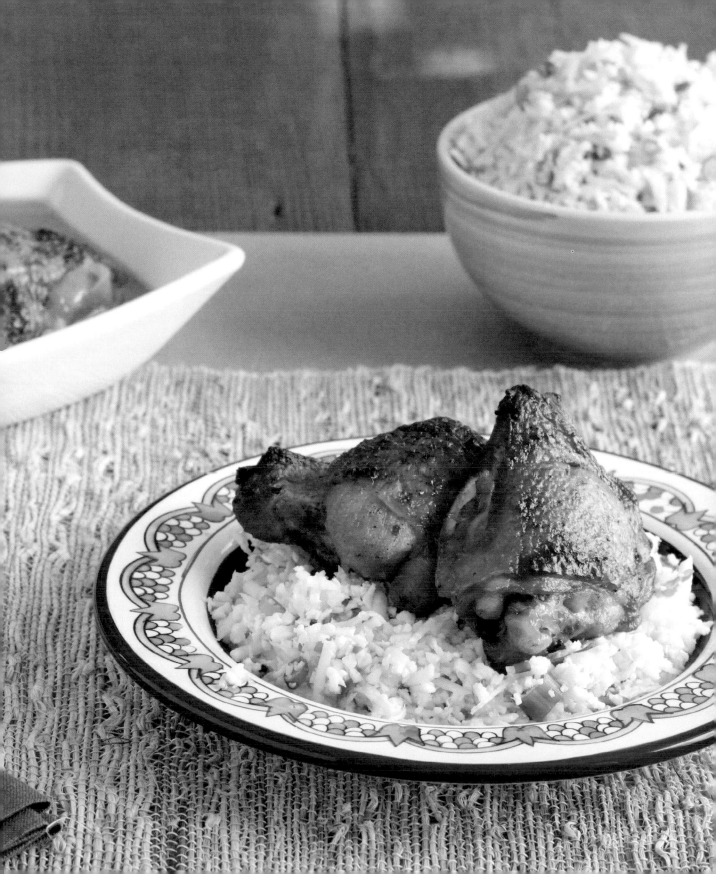

lemon ginger chicken

PREP TIME **10 MINS** • COOK TIME **20 TO 25 MINS** • SERVINGS **4**

NUTS

EGGS

NIGHTSHADES

FODMAPS

SEAFOOD

1/4 cup coconut aminos*

1/2 teaspoon ground ginger

1/4 teaspoon sea salt

1/4 teaspoon black pepper

1 lemon, cut in half

2 teaspoons arrowroot flour

2 pounds boneless, skinless chicken thighs

2 tablespoons coconut oil or ghee

8 green onions (scallions), sliced (1 cup)

1 tablespoon sesame seeds, plus more for garnish

1 teaspoon cold-pressed sesame oil, to finish

Asian Sautéed Greens, for serving (page 140)

Preheat the oven to 350°F.

Marinate the chicken: In a large mixing bowl, whisk together the coconut aminos, ginger, salt, pepper, juice of half the lemon, and arrowroot flour. Place the chicken in the bowl and turn to coat in the marinade; let marinate for 5 minutes.

Heat the coconut oil in a large oven-safe skillet over medium heat. While the pan is heating, cut the remaining lemon half into slices. When the oil is hot, carefully place the chicken in the pan and cook it for 2 minutes per side. Pour the marinade over the chicken; top with the green onions, sesame seeds, and lemon slices. Place the pan in the oven and bake for 15 to 20 minutes or until the chicken is cooked through (no pink remains) and reaches an internal temperature of 165°F.

Garnish with a drizzle of sesame oil and more sesame seeds.

Serve with Asian Sautéed Greens.

INGREDIENT TIP
*Check out pages 226–227 for a list of recommended brands. ●

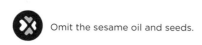
Omit the sesame oil and seeds.

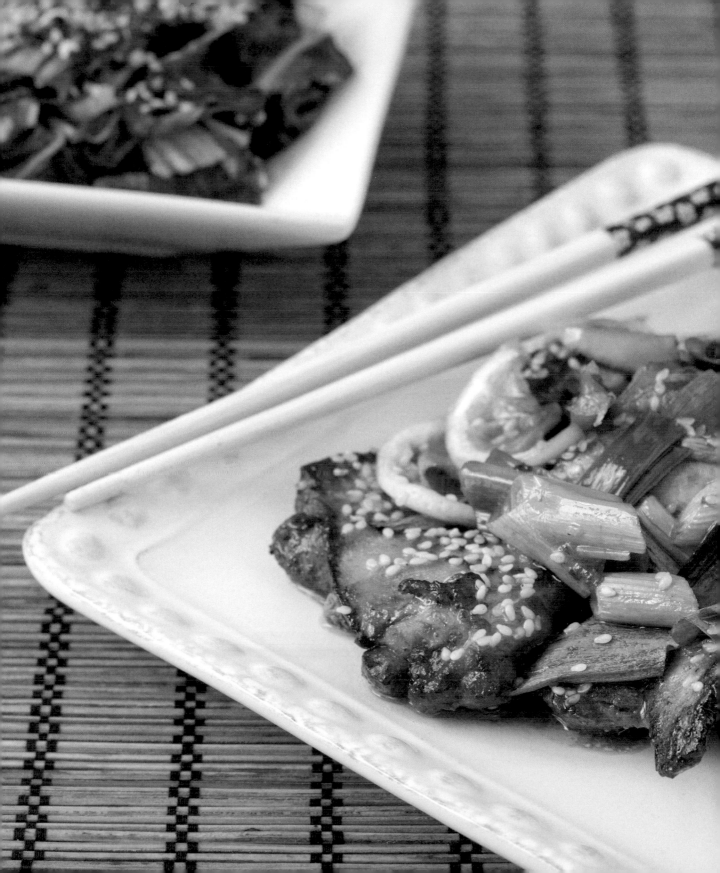

tandoori chicken skewers

PREP TIME **20 MINS (+ 3 OR MORE HRS TO MARINATE)** • COOK TIME **20 MINS**

• SERVINGS **6 TO 8**

NUTS

EGGS

NIGHTSHADES

FODMAPS

SEAFOOD

3/4 cup full-fat coconut milk, canned* or homemade (page 210)

1/2 small red onion, chopped

3 cloves garlic

1 teaspoon ground ginger

2 tablespoons tomato paste

2 teaspoons ground coriander

1 teaspoon ground cumin

1 teaspoon paprika

1/2 teaspoon sea salt

4 boneless, skinless chicken breasts (2 pounds total), cut into 1 1/2-inch cubes

skewers for grilling (see Kitchen Tip)

Combine all the ingredients except the chicken cubes in a blender or food processor and process for 1 to 2 minutes or until the marinade is creamy. Place the chicken in a large plastic zip-top bag or container and pour the coconut milk mixture over the chicken. Refrigerate for at least 3 hours or overnight.

When you are ready to cook the chicken, preheat a grill or grill pan to high heat. While you are waiting for the grill to heat up, put 5 to 6 cubes of chicken on each skewer. Reduce the heat to medium and place the skewers on the grill. Grill for 8 to 10 minutes and then turn each skewer over—you know the skewer is ready to be flipped when the chicken releases easily from the grates. Grill each skewer for another 10 to 12 minutes or until cooked through, so no pink is visible on the inside, and the chicken reaches an internal temperature of 165°F.

These skewers pair perfectly with the Moroccan Cauli-Rice Pilaf on page 137 and the Mini Sweet Potato Flatbreads (for Energy Modifications) on page 156.

INGREDIENT TIP
*Check out pages 226–227 for a list of recommended brands.

KITCHEN TIP
If using wooden skewers, soak them in water for at least 15 minutes to keep them from burning on the grill. ●

Make this with swordfish or a similar-texture fish and marinate for just 15 to 20 minutes.

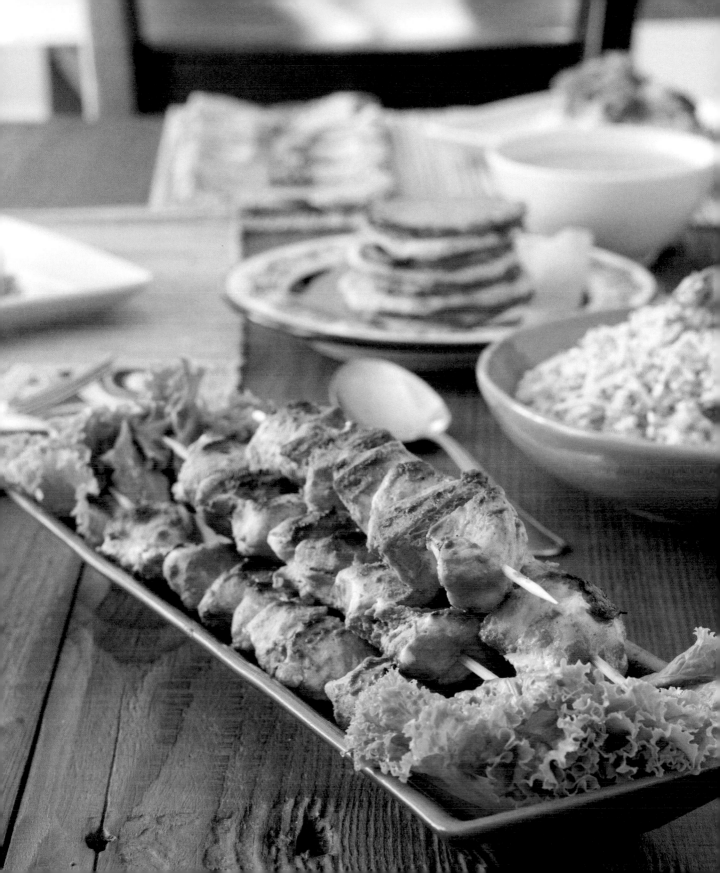

zoodles with creamy tomato sauce & chicken

PREP TIME **15 MINS (+ MARINARA AND CHICKEN PREP)** • COOK TIME **15 MINS** • SERVINGS **4**

NUTS

EGGS

NIGHTSHADES

FODMAPS

SEAFOOD

4 large or 8 small zucchini, yellow squash, or a combination

1 recipe Simple Marinara (page 217)

1/4 cup full-fat coconut milk, canned* or homemade (page 210)

2 large boneless, skinless chicken breasts (about 1 pound total), cooked (see Chef Note)

Fill a large pot with 1 inch of water, cover, and bring to a boil over high heat. Place a steamer basket in the pot.

While the water comes to a boil, shred the zucchini or yellow squash into noodles using a handheld julienne peeler, a spiralizer tool, or even a regular vegetable peeler (if using a regular peeler, the noodles will be wide and flat instead of spaghetti-shaped). You should get 4 cups of noodles. When the water is boiling, steam the noodles in the basket for 3 minutes, then place them in a colander to drain off the excess liquid as they cool slightly.

In a large skillet over low heat, warm the Simple Marinara and coconut milk. Reheat your chicken if using leftovers.

Once the sauce is hot, add the zoodles to the sauce and toss to combine. Slice the chicken into thin strips and serve on top of the zoodles and sauce. You may also chop up some smaller pieces to incorporate throughout the dish.

INGREDIENT TIP
*Check out pages 226–227 for a list of recommended brands.

CHEF NOTE
If you don't have sufficient leftover chicken on hand for this recipe, simply season boneless, skinless chicken breasts with sea salt and black pepper and bake in a 350°F oven until done, or use breast meat from a clean-ingredient store-bought rotisserie chicken. ●

 Make this with cooked shrimp instead of chicken.

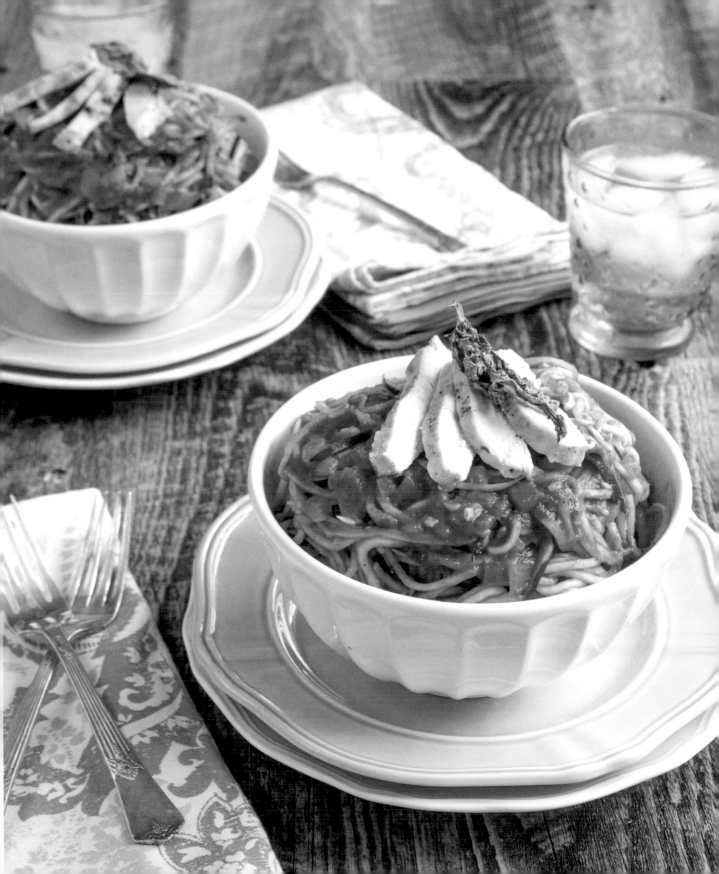

chicken strips

PREP TIME **15 MINS** • COOK TIME **35 TO 40 MINS** • SERVINGS **4 TO 6**

NUTS

EGGS

NIGHTSHADES

FODMAPS

SEAFOOD

1 cup arrowroot flour

1 cup almond flour*

2 teaspoons black pepper

4 teaspoons granulated garlic

1 1/2 teaspoons sea salt

1/2 teaspoon paprika

1/2 cup full-fat coconut milk, canned* or homemade (page 210)

2 tablespoons hot sauce*

4 boneless, skinless chicken breasts (about 1 1/2 to 2 pounds total), cut into 1-inch strips

1/2 cup coconut oil, melted

BBQ Sauce (page 199), Sweetener-Free Ketchup (page 216), or No-Honey Mustard Sauce (page 202), for serving

Preheat the oven to 400°F. Line a rimmed baking sheet with parchment paper.

In a wide, shallow bowl or dish, mix together the arrowroot flour, almond flour, pepper, granulated garlic, salt, and paprika. Combine the coconut milk and hot sauce in another wide, shallow bowl or dish.

Pat each chicken strip dry with a paper towel. Dip each strip in the coconut milk mixture, shaking off the excess. Gently place the strip in the dry mixture and coat heavily. Place each coated chicken strip on the prepared baking sheet and bake for 20 minutes. Using a pastry or sauce brush, gently pat the top of each strip with the melted coconut oil. Continue baking for another 15 to 20 minutes or until the chicken is no longer pink in the center.

Serve with BBQ Sauce, Sweetener-Free Ketchup, or No-Honey Mustard Sauce.

INGREDIENT TIP
*Check out pages 226–227 for a list of recommended brands. ●

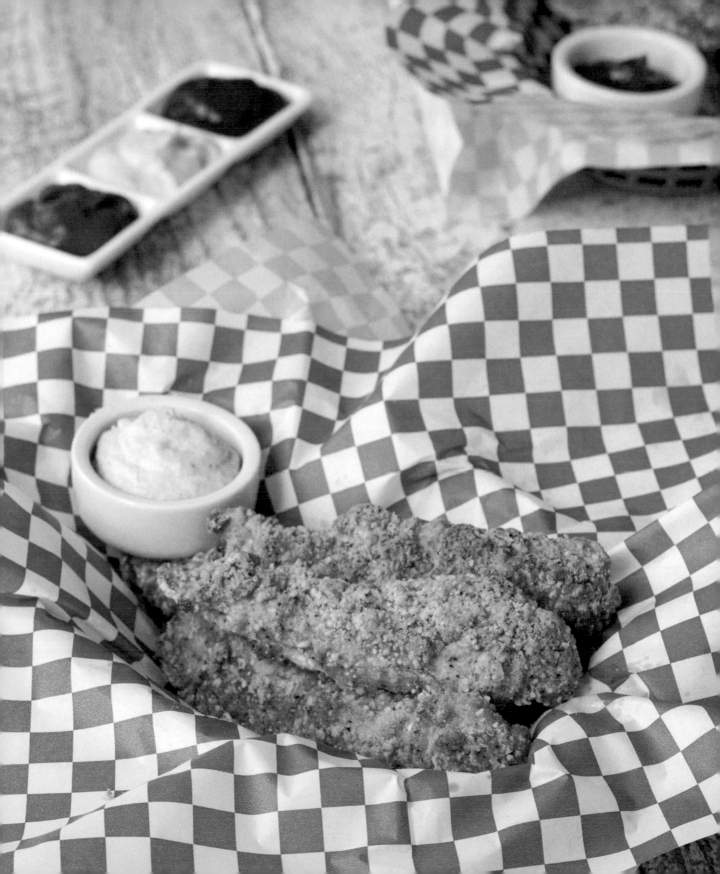

NUTS

EGGS

NIGHTSHADES

FODMAPS

SEAFOOD

curried chicken salad with apples

PREP TIME **20 MINS** • SERVINGS **4 TO 6**

1 cup Healthy Homemade
Mayonnaise (page 219)

3 tablespoons apple cider
vinegar*

3 tablespoons yellow curry
powder

4 boneless, skinless chicken
breasts (about 2 pounds
total), cooked, cooled, and
diced

1/2 medium red onion, diced

3 green onions (scallions),
sliced

3 celery stalks, sliced

2 green apples, diced

FOR SERVING
cucumber slices, green
apple slices, jicama slices,
avocado slices, and/or
mixed greens

INGREDIENT TIP
*Check out pages
226–227 for a list
of recommended
brands. ●

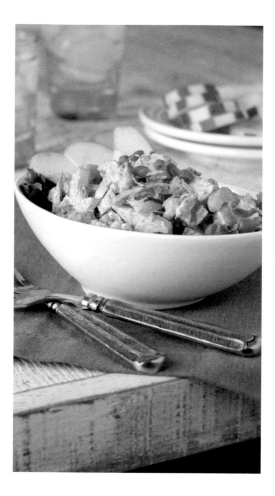

Mix the Mayonnaise and apple cider vinegar in a small bowl. Sprinkle the curry powder over the mayonnaise mixture and whisk until evenly distributed. In a large bowl, combine the chicken, red onion, green onions, celery, and apples. Pour the mayonnaise mixture over the chicken and stir until evenly coated.

Serve with your choice of accompaniment.

 Make this with canned tuna or salmon instead of chicken.*

bbq chicken

PREP TIME **5 MINS** • COOK TIME **25 TO 30 MINS** • SERVINGS **4**

4 bone-in, skin-on chicken leg quarters or 8 chicken legs and/or thighs

sea salt and black pepper

2 cups BBQ Sauce (page 199)

NUTS

EGGS

NIGHTSHADES

FODMAPS

SEAFOOD

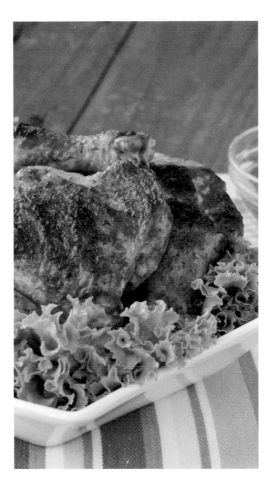

Preheat a grill or grill pan to high heat. Rinse the chicken and pat dry.

Reduce the heat to medium. Season the chicken generously on both sides with salt and pepper and place the chicken on the grill skin-side down. Cook the chicken for 10 minutes, then flip the pieces over and baste with the BBQ Sauce. Cook for another 15 to 20 minutes or until the internal temperature reaches 165°F,

basting every couple of minutes with the BBQ Sauce. If you're having trouble getting the chicken to cook through while keeping the sauce from burning, transfer it into a preheated 350°F oven on a rimmed sheet pan or onto a grill pan to finish cooking through.

Serve with more BBQ Sauce for dipping.

NUTS

EGGS

NIGHTSHADES

FODMAPS

SEAFOOD

beef & bacon cottage pie

PREP TIME **15 MINS** • COOK TIME **50 MINS** • SERVINGS **6**

1 medium butternut squash (2 1/2 pounds)

2 tablespoons ghee or coconut oil

sea salt and black pepper

8 slices bacon, cut into 1/2-inch pieces, plus more for garnish if desired

2 medium carrots, diced (1 cup)

1 cup diced green beans

1/2 medium yellow onion, diced (1 cup)

2 pounds ground beef or bison

4 tablespoons Smoky Spice Blend (page 222)

Preheat the oven to 375°F.

Peel the butternut squash with a vegetable peeler and cut in half lengthwise. Remove the seeds and chop into 1-inch pieces. Set up a pot with 1 to 2 inches of water and a steamer basket. Steam the squash over high heat until fork-tender, about 15 to 20 minutes. While still warm, transfer the squash to a food processor and blend with the ghee, seasoning with salt and pepper to taste.

While the squash is steaming, cook the bacon in a large skillet over medium heat until the fat has rendered off, about 8 to 10 minutes. Remove the bacon from the skillet with a slotted spoon and set aside, leaving the bacon fat in the pan. Add the carrots and green beans to the skillet and cook for 5 minutes over medium heat. Add the onion and continue cooking until the carrots just begin soften, about 5 more minutes. Crumble the ground meat into the pan and sprinkle with the Spice Blend; use a spatula to break up any clumps of meat and to mix the meat and Spice Blend together. Cook until the meat is just browned and the carrots are cooked through.

Transfer the meat mixture to an oven-safe baking dish, either a deep pie plate or a 9-by-13-inch rectangular dish. Arrange the bacon pieces on top of the meat, reserving a small handful for garnish, then top with a layer of the butternut squash puree. Bake for 20 minutes or until the top just starts to brown. Garnish with extra bacon.

 Use cooked and mashed sweet potatoes instead of butternut squash as the topping.

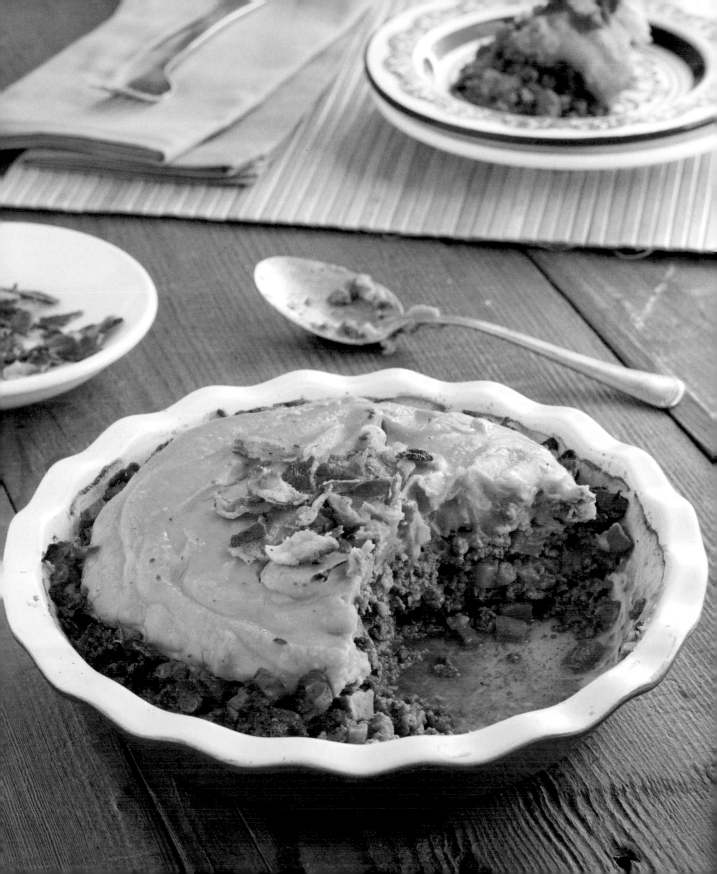

cinnamon & fennel braised pork

PREP TIME **15 MINS** • COOK TIME **8+ HRS** • SERVINGS **8**

NUTS

EGGS

NIGHTSHADES

FODMAPS

SEAFOOD

2 green apples, peeled and roughly chopped

1 fennel bulb, roughly chopped (save fronds for garnish)

1 small yellow onion, roughly chopped

4 cloves garlic, roughly chopped

2 tablespoons ground cinnamon

1 teaspoon sea salt

1 teaspoon black pepper

1/2 teaspoon ground cumin

1 teaspoon gluten-free brown mustard*

4 tablespoons apple cider vinegar,* divided

2 tablespoons bacon fat or coconut oil

1 (3-pound) pork roast, such as shoulder or butt

1/2 cup water

2 cinnamon sticks

Place the apples, fennel, onion, and garlic in the bottom of a slow cooker. In a small mixing bowl, mix together the ground cinnamon, salt, pepper, cumin, mustard, and 1 tablespoon of apple cider vinegar to form a paste. Spread the bacon fat over the top of the pork, then spread the spice paste over the top and sides of the meat. Carefully place the pork on top of the vegetables in the slow cooker. Add the remaining 3 tablespoons of apple cider vinegar, water, and cinnamon sticks to the bottom of the slow cooker.

Cook on low for 8 hours or until the meat is tender and pulls apart easily with a fork. Garnish with the reserved fennel fronds if desired.

INGREDIENT TIP

*Check out pages 226–227 for a list of recommended brands.

KITCHEN TIP

No slow cooker? No problem! Cook this dish in an enameled cast-iron Dutch oven at 200°F for 8 hours or until the meat is tender and pulls apart easily with a fork. ●

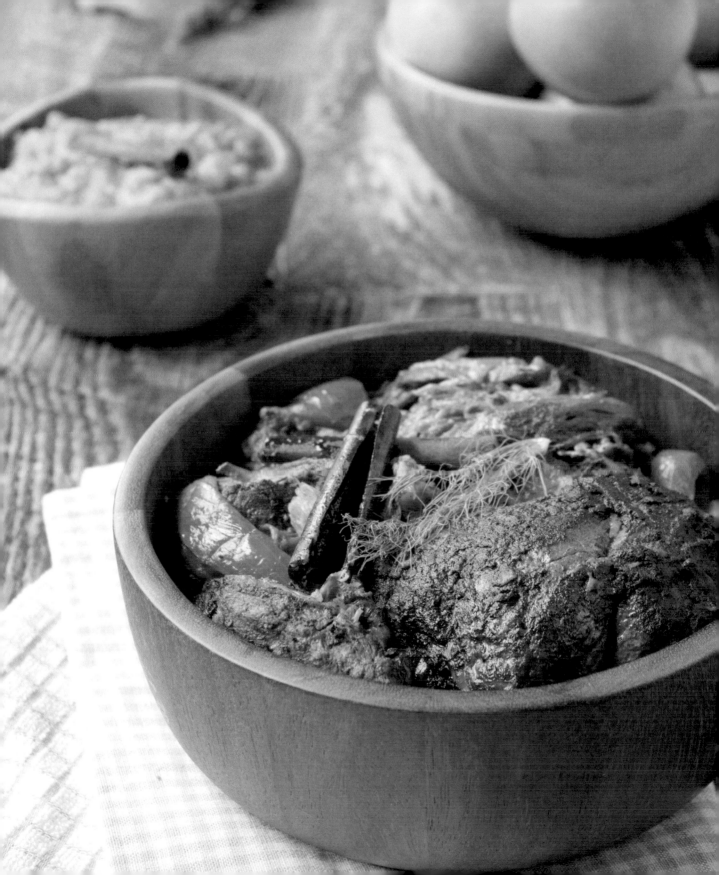

MAIN
DISHES

NUTS

EGGS

NIGHTSHADES

FODMAPS

SEAFOOD

fennel & sage meatballs

PREP TIME **20 MINS** • COOK TIME **40 MINS** • SERVINGS **5**

FOR SERVING
1 spaghetti squash (optional)

FOR THE MEATBALLS
2 pounds ground beef, bison, or a mixture
2 tablespoons minced fresh sage
1 teaspoon ground coriander
1 teaspoon ground cumin
1 teaspoon sea salt
1/4 teaspoon black pepper

FOR THE SAUCE
1 tablespoon coconut oil
1 medium yellow onion, diced (about 2 cups)
1 fennel bulb, diced (about 2 cups)
1 teaspoon ground coriander
1 teaspoon ground cumin
1 teaspoon sea salt
1 (6-ounce) can tomato paste
1 (14.5-oz) can diced tomatoes
1 1/2 cups water
2 tablespoons minced fresh sage

Preheat the oven to 375°F.

Make the spaghetti squash, if using: Cut the spaghetti squash in half lengthwise and remove the seeds and inner membranes, then sprinkle liberally with salt and pepper. Place the squash halves facedown on a baking sheet. Roast for approximately 40 minutes or until the skin gives when you press on it and the "noodles" inside release easily from the skin. Use a fork to remove the noodles.

While the squash bakes, make the meatballs: Place the ground meat in a large bowl and sprinkle the rest of the meatball ingredients on top. Mix with your hands to thoroughly combine the seasonings. Use about 2 tablespoons of the mixture to form each meatball and set aside.

Make the sauce: In a large saucepan over medium-high heat, melt the coconut oil. Add the onion and fennel and cook until soft, about 5 minutes. Sprinkle the coriander, cumin, and salt over the onion mixture and mix well. Add the tomato paste, diced tomatoes, and water and stir until well combined. Mix in the minced sage.

Bring the sauce to a boil and then gently drop in the meatballs. Reduce the heat to medium-low, cover the pan, and simmer for about 20 minutes, gently turning the meatballs about halfway through.

Serve over spaghetti squash.

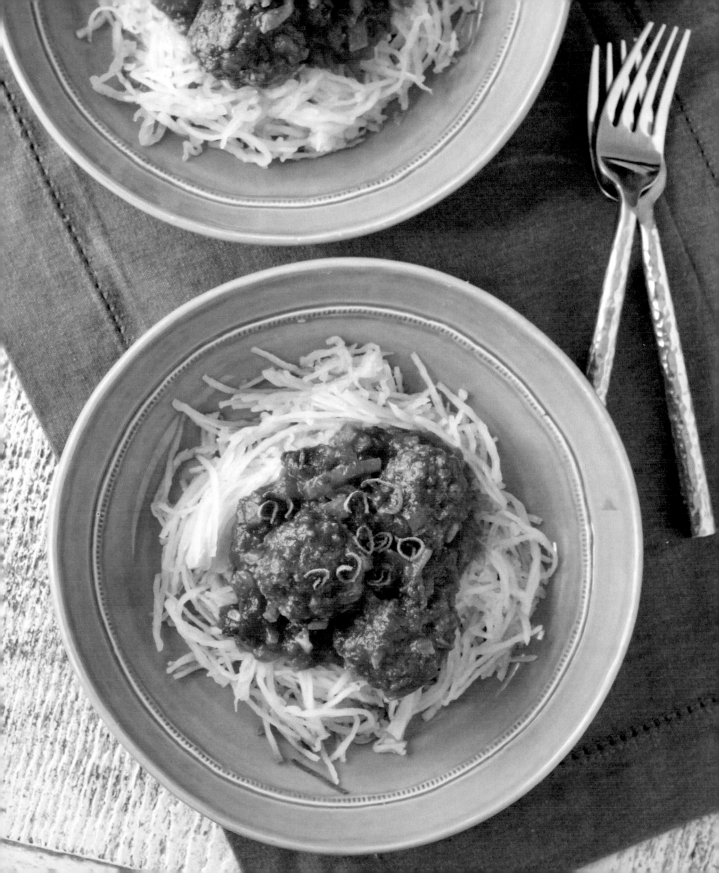

asian ginger flank steak

PREP TIME **10 MINS (+ 3 HRS TO MARINATE)** • COOK TIME **18 MINS** • SERVINGS **4 TO 6**

1 tablespoon Garlic Chili Paste (page 196)

zest of 1 lemon (1 tablespoon)

1 (2-inch) piece of fresh ginger, minced or grated (2 tablespoons)

2 tablespoons minced or grated garlic

1/2 cup coconut aminos*

1/4 teaspoon sea salt

1 to 1 1/2 pounds flank steak

1/4 cup cold-pressed sesame oil

Spicy Slaw (page 134), for serving

Combine all the ingredients except the flank steak, sesame oil, and slaw in a bowl. Put the flank steak in a plastic zip-top bag and pour the marinade ingredients over it, making sure the meat is evenly coated. Push all the air out of the bag and seal it. Refrigerate for at least 3 hours.

Preheat a grill or grill pan to high heat. Remove the steak from the bag and dispose of the leftover marinade. Place the steak on the grill and cook for 8 minutes before flipping. Cook for an additional 8 to 10 minutes, depending on the desired level of doneness. Remove from the heat and let sit, covered, for 10 minutes before slicing and serving.

Drizzle the steak slices with the sesame oil and serve with Spicy Slaw.

INGREDIENT TIP
*Check out pages 226–227 for a list of recommended brands. ●

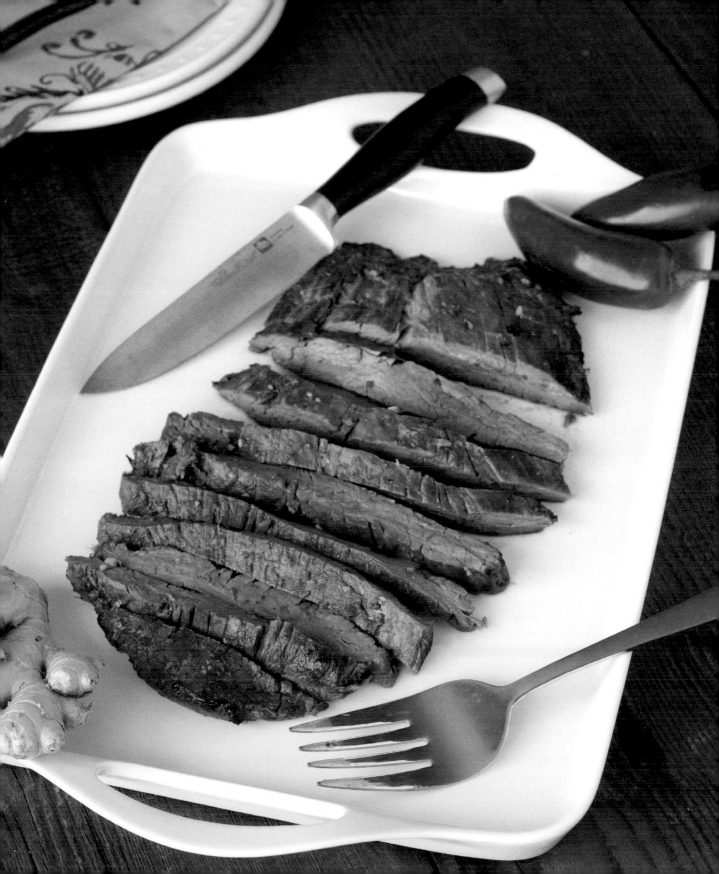

beef larb (thai lettuce wraps)

PREP TIME **20 MINS** • COOK TIME **10 TO 12 MINS** • SERVINGS **4**

NUTS

EGGS

NIGHTSHADES

FODMAPS

SEAFOOD

FOR THE FILLING

juice of 1 lime

2 tablespoons coconut aminos*

1 tablespoon fish sauce*

1 stalk lemongrass

1 tablespoon cooking fat**

2 shallots, minced (2/3 cup)

2 cloves garlic, minced

2 Thai red chilie peppers or other spicy red chili peppers, very thinly sliced, plus more for garnish if desired

zest of 2 limes

1 1/2 pounds ground beef (or other ground meat/ shrimp)

FOR THE SAUCE

juice of 2 limes

2 tablespoons fish sauce*

1 tablespoon Garlic Chili Paste (page 196)

1 large head butter lettuce, separated into individual leaves

OPTIONAL GARNISHES

1/2 cup chopped fresh mint and/or cilantro

1 lime, cut into wedges to squeeze over the wraps

Making the filling: In a small bowl, whisk together the lime juice, coconut aminos, and fish sauce. Set aside. Trim the base (the white end) off the lemongrass as well as the top third or half of the green part, leaving a 4-inch piece. Then peel off any dry or tough outer layers and mince the lemongrass. In a large skillet over medium heat, melt the cooking fat. Add the shallots and garlic and cook for 1 minute. Add the chilie peppers, lemongrass, and lime zest and cook for about 30 seconds or until fragrant. Crumble the ground beef into the skillet and continue to cook for about 5 to 8 minutes until cooked through, stirring to break it up and allow it to brown evenly. Pour the lime juice mixture over the meat, stir to incorporate, and cook for an additional 1 minute.

Make the sauce: In small bowl, whisk together the lime juice, fish sauce, and Garlic Chili Paste.

Serve the meat in a butter lettuce leaf, top with the sauce, and garnish with mint or cilantro and lime wedges, if using.

INGREDIENT TIP
*Check out pages 226–227 for a list of recommended brands.

CHEF NOTE
**See page 228 for recommended cooking fats.

SEAFOOD-FREE?
Omit the fish sauce. ●

 Make this with chopped/ground shrimp instead of beef.

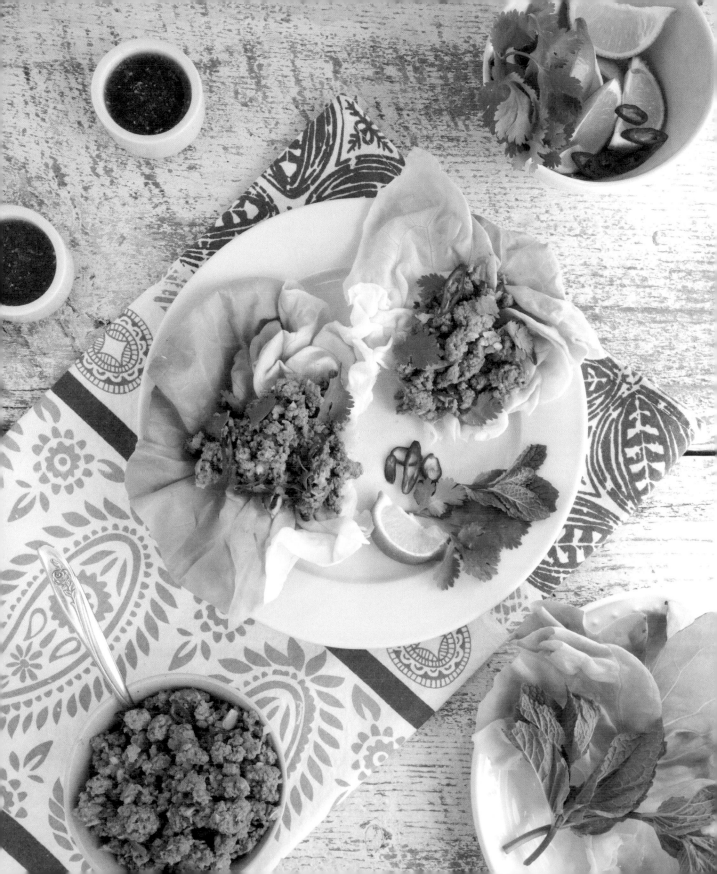

pot roast with root veggies & mushrooms

PREP TIME **15 MINS** • COOK TIME **8+ HRS** • SERVINGS **4**

NUTS

EGGS

NIGHTSHADES

FODMAPS

SEAFOOD

....

1 tablespoon cooking fat*

1/2 teaspoon onion powder

1/2 teaspoon granulated garlic

1 teaspoon sea salt

1 teaspoon black pepper

1 1/2 pounds bottom round roast

1 1/2 cups Bone Broth, beef with garlic (page 208)

1 medium onion, sliced

2 extra-large carrots, chopped (3 to 4 cups)

1 large parsnip, chopped (1 1/2 cups)

6 to 8 mushrooms, quartered

1 tablespoon apple cider vinegar** or balsamic vinegar

1 large sprig fresh rosemary, plus more for garnish if desired

1/2 teaspoon dried thyme

OPTIONAL ADDITIONS

1/2 cup Sweetener-Free Ketchup (page 216) or crushed or diced tomatoes (omit for nightshade-free)

1 green apple, peeled and chopped

In a cast-iron or stainless-steel skillet over high heat, melt the cooking fat. While the pan heats up, combine the onion powder, granulated garlic, salt, and pepper in a small bowl, then season the meat liberally on all sides with the spice mixture. Sear the meat in the skillet for 2 minutes on each side. Place the seared meat in a slow cooker along with the Bone Broth, onion, carrots, parsnip, mushrooms, vinegar, and herbs. Add the Ketchup, crushed or diced tomatoes, or apple, if using.

Cook on low for 8 hours or more, until the meat comes apart easily with a fork.

To make a quick gravy: When the meat is done cooking, pour the remaining liquid and 1/2 cup of the cooked carrots and parsnips into a blender and purée on high for 1 to 2 minutes or until smooth.

CHEF NOTES
*See page 228 for recommended cooking fats.

Pot roast tastes great with Thousand Island Dressing (page 204) or a gluten-free mustard.*

INGREDIENT TIP
**Check out pages 226–227 for a list of recommended brands. ●

 Do not use the optional ketchup or tomatoes.

 Use 1 large sweet potato, peeled and diced, instead of the carrots.

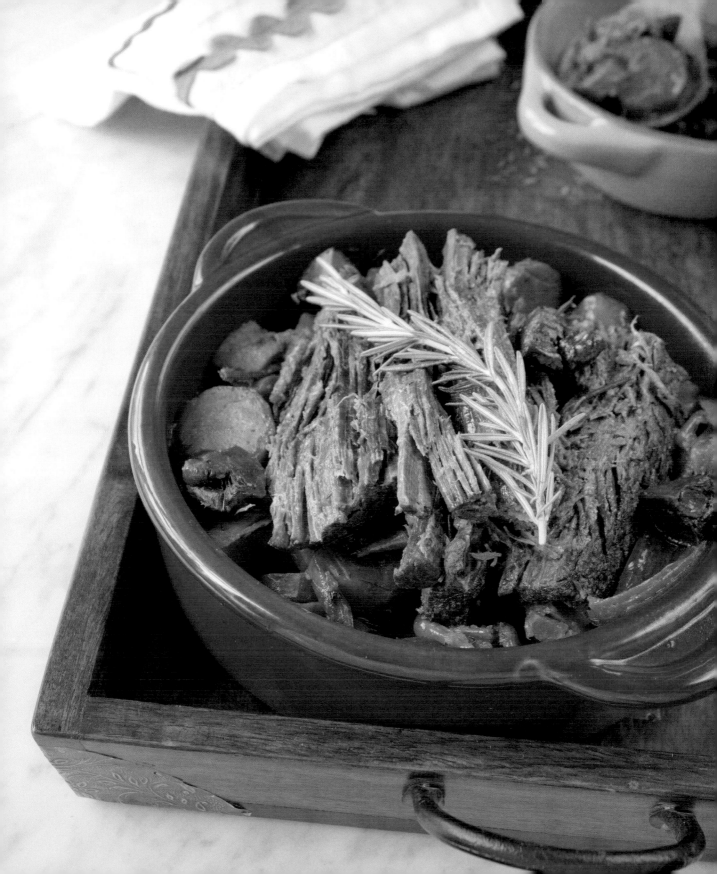

satay skewers

**PREP TIME 15 MINS (+ 30 MINS TO MARINATE) • COOK TIME 10 TO 15 MINS
• SERVINGS 4**

NUTS
EGGS
NIGHTSHADES
FODMAPS
SEAFOOD

FOR THE MARINADE
1/2 large stalk lemongrass, sliced (2 tablespoons)
1/4 cup sliced shallots
2 cloves garlic, minced
pinch of red pepper flakes
1/4 to 1/2 teaspoon minced fresh ginger
1 teaspoon ground turmeric
1 teaspoon ground coriander
1 teaspoon ground cumin
3 tablespoons coconut aminos*
3 to 6 tablespoons fish sauce*
1 cardamom pod, smashed
1/4 cup full-fat coconut milk, canned* or homemade (page 210)
sea salt and black pepper
1 1/2 pounds flank steak

FOR THE SAUCE
3 tablespoons almond butter*
1/4 cup coconut aminos*
1 tablespoon full-fat coconut milk, canned* or homemade (page 210)
5 to 6 drops fish sauce*
1/2 teaspoon onion powder
12–18 wooden skewers

1/4 cup chopped fresh cilantro, for garnish
1 lime, cut into wedges, for garnish

Soak 12 to 18 wooden skewers in water in a shallow dish.

Make the marinade: Mix together all the marinade ingredients in a mixing bowl.

Slice the steak against the grain into 1/2-inch strips. Place the steak in the bowl with the marinade and toss to combine. Marinate for 30 minutes.

Make the sauce: Whisk together all the sauce ingredients in a small mixing bowl.

Preheat a grill or grill pan to medium-high heat. Lace each strip of steak onto a skewer, and place the skewers on the hot grill. Cook the skewers in batches for 2 to 3 minutes per side, flipping once. Repeat until all of the skewers are cooked. Garnish with cilantro and lime wedges and serve with the sauce.

INGREDIENT TIP
*Check out pages 226–227 for a list of recommended brands.

NUT FREE?
Use sesame tahini or Sunbutter (page 164) instead of almond butter.

NIGHTSHADE FREE?
Omit the red pepper flakes.

SEAFOOD FREE?
Omit the fish sauce. ●

Make this with shrimp instead of beef.

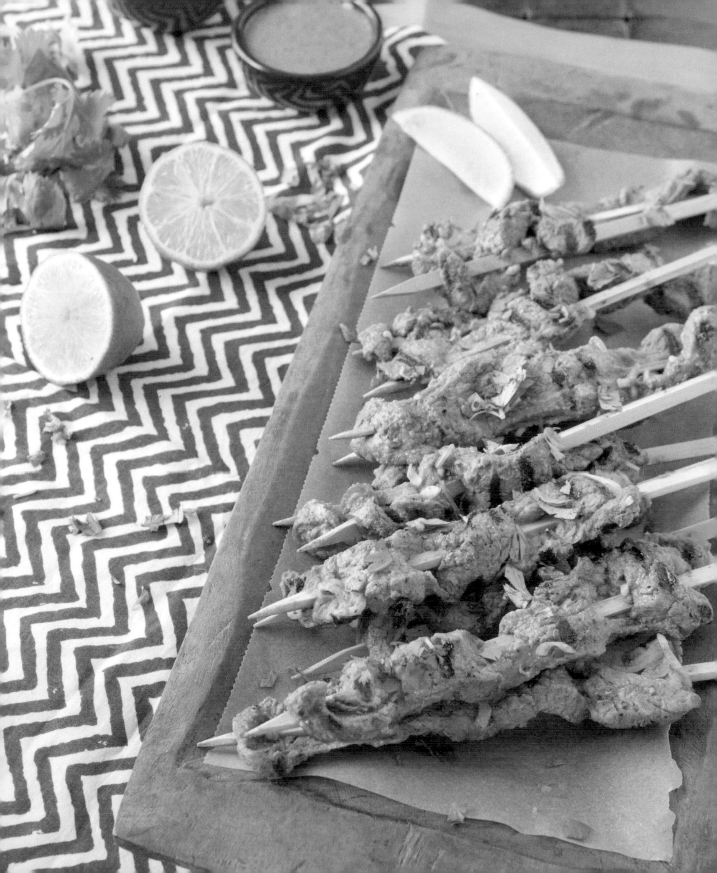

10-minute sliders

PREP TIME **4 MINS** • COOK TIME **6 MINS** • SERVINGS **4**

NUTS

EGGS

NIGHTSHADES

FODMAPS

SEAFOOD

1 teaspoon granulated garlic

2 teaspoons onion powder

1/2 teaspoon sea salt

1/2 teaspoon black pepper

1/2 teaspoon ground cumin (optional)

1 1/2 pounds ground beef, bison, or lamb

1/2 head iceberg lettuce

1 tomato, sliced (optional, omit for nightshade free)

1/2 red onion, sliced

Creamy Ranch Dressing (page 204), for serving (optional, omit for egg free)

Preheat a large cast-iron skillet, grill, or grill pan to medium-high heat.

Combine the garlic, onion powder, salt, pepper, and cumin in a small bowl. Form the meat into 8 small (3-ounce) patties, taking care not to overhandle the meat or it will become tough. Use your thumb to imprint a small dent into the center of each patty. With clean hands, liberally season both sides of the patties with the Spice Blend, using a utensil to flip the patties so that your hands do not get dirty between dips into the spices. There may be extra spice left over; it can be stored in a jar for later use.

Cook the patties for 3 minutes per side or until they reach the desired level of doneness.

Serve over iceberg lettuce, topped with tomato and onion slices or with your favorite burger toppings. These sliders are perfect when topped with Creamy Ranch Dressing.

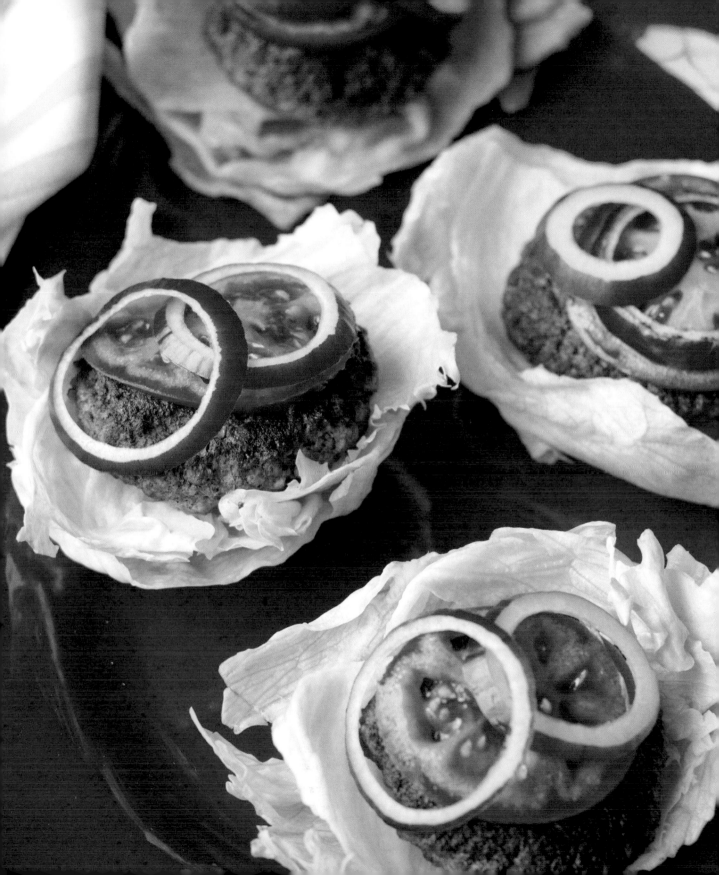

chorizo burgers with
spicy red onions

PREP TIME **10 MINS** • COOK TIME **15 TO 20 MINS** • SERVINGS **4**

NUTS

EGGS

NIGHTSHADES

FODMAPS

SEAFOOD

3 tablespoons ghee or coconut oil, plus more for the squash

1 red onion, sliced

3 tablespoons Chorizo Spice Blend (page 222), divided

1 1/2 pounds ground beef or bison (or a blend)

4 (1/4-inch-thick) slices butternut squash, peeled (optional)

sea salt

mixed greens or lettuce and additional toppings of your choice, such as avocado, tomato, and bacon, for serving

Preheat a grill or grill pan to medium heat.

Heat the ghee or coconut oil in a skillet over medium heat. Sauté the onion in the skillet for about 10 minutes, until soft. Sprinkle 1 tablespoon of the Spice Blend over the onion and cook for another 2 to 3 minutes.

In a bowl, combine the meat with the remaining 2 tablespoons of the Spice Blend. Form into 4 patties. Grill the burgers over medium heat for about 5 minutes per side or to the desired doneness.

Brush the butternut squash slices with ghee or coconut oil and sprinkle with sea salt. Grill each side for about 3 minutes or until just cooked through.

To serve, place the burgers over mixed greens or lettuce and top with the butternut squash rings, onions, and any additional toppings of your choice.

These burgers pair well with Seasoned Sweet Potato Fries, page 160.

 Pair with Seasoned Sweet Potato Fries on page 160.

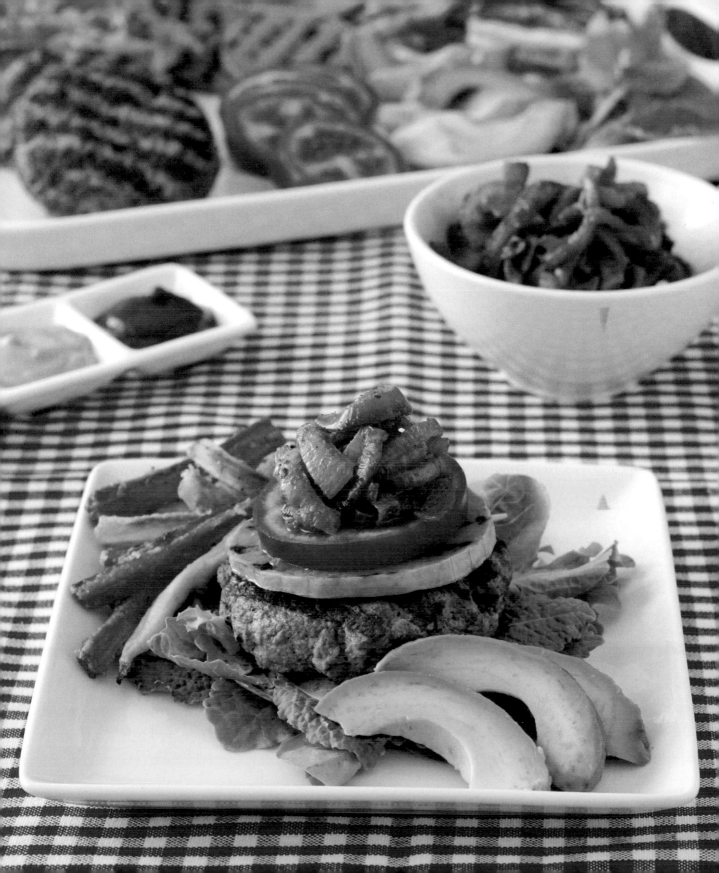

coffee & cocoa rubbed ribs

PREP TIME **10 MINS (+ 3 HRS TO MARINATE)** • COOK TIME **3 1/2 HRS** • SERVINGS **6**

NUTS

EGGS

NIGHTSHADES

FODMAPS

SEAFOOD

FOR THE RUB

2 tablespoons finely ground coffee beans

1 1/2 tablespoons sea salt

1 tablespoon paprika

1 tablespoon ancho chili powder

1 teaspoon granulated garlic

1 teaspoon onion powder

1 teaspoon black pepper

1 teaspoon unsweetened cocoa powder*

2 racks St. Louis style pork ribs (about 5 to 6 pounds total)

1 cup BBQ Sauce (page 199, optional)

To make the rub, combine all the dry ingredients in a small bowl. Coat both sides of each rack of ribs with the rub, wrap tightly with foil, and refrigerate for at least 3 hours, preferably overnight.

Preheat the oven to 275°F. Remove the ribs from the refrigerator and, keeping them foil-wrapped, place them in the oven on a rimmed baking sheet, foil seam up. Cook for 2 to 3 hours or until the rib meat easily separates from the bone. Remove from the oven and unwrap from the foil.

Place the oven rack in the top position and preheat the broiler to high, or preheat a grill or grill pan to high. If using BBQ Sauce, coat each rack with the sauce. Place the rack of ribs in the oven on a rimmed baking sheet or directly on the grill and cook for an additional 5 minutes or until the outsides of the ribs are crispy.

Serve plain or with BBQ Sauce.

INGREDIENT TIP

*Check out pages 226–227 for a list of recommended brands.

CHEF NOTE

These ribs are even better the next day so make them ahead of time if you can. ●

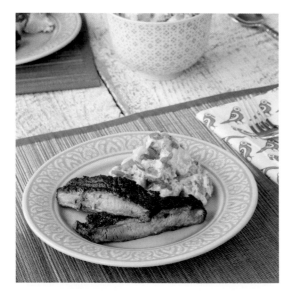

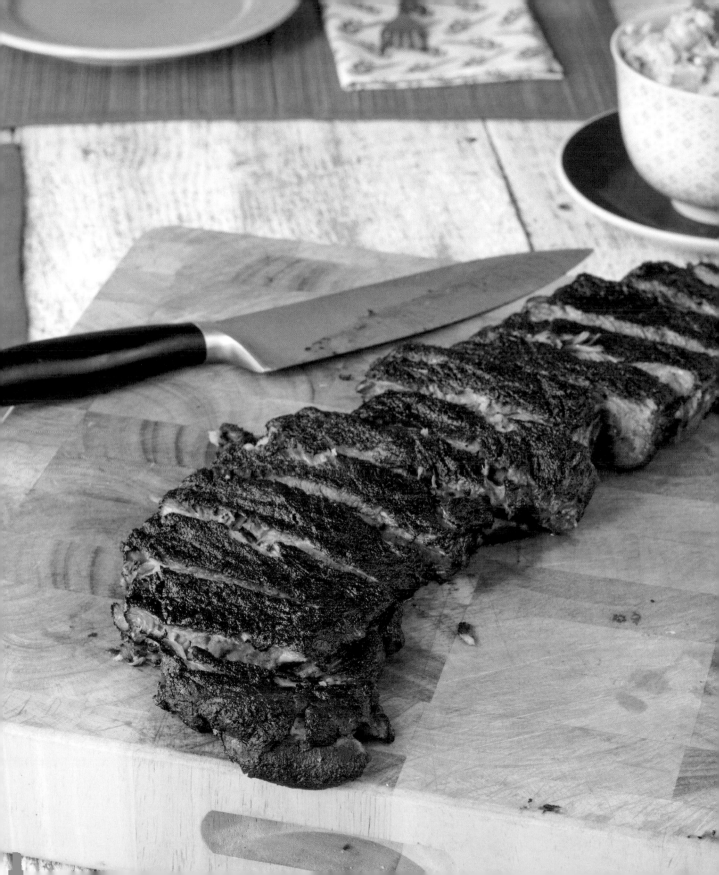

lamb burgers with chunky avo-ziki

PREP TIME **20 MINS** • COOK TIME **8 TO 12 MINS** • SERVINGS **4**

NUTS
EGGS
NIGHTSHADES
FODMAPS
SEAFOOD

1/2 teaspoon sea salt

1/2 teaspoon black pepper

1/2 teaspoon dried oregano

1 teaspoon chopped fresh dill

1 clove garlic, minced

zest of 1 lemon (optional)

1 1/2 pounds ground lamb

FOR THE AVO-ZIKI

2 ripe avocados, mashed with a fork

1/2 cup grated cucumber

1 teaspoon chopped fresh dill

2 cloves garlic, minced

juice of 2 lemons

2 tablespoons extra-virgin olive oil

sea salt and black pepper to taste

FOR SERVING

1/2 head iceberg lettuce, separated into leaves

4 large tomato slices (optional, omit for nightshade-free)

8 slices cucumber

8 thin slices red onion

Make the burgers: Preheat a grill or grill pan to medium-high heat. In a mixing bowl, combine the salt, pepper, oregano, dill, garlic, and lemon zest, if using. Add the meat and mix with your hands until well incorporated. Form the mixture into 4 patties, then grill for 4 to 5 minutes per side (depending on thickness) to your desired level of doneness.

Make the avo-ziki: Combine all the ingredients in a small mixing bowl.

Serve the burgers in lettuce wraps topped with tomato, cucumber, onion slices, and avo-ziki.

 Do not use the optional tomato slices.

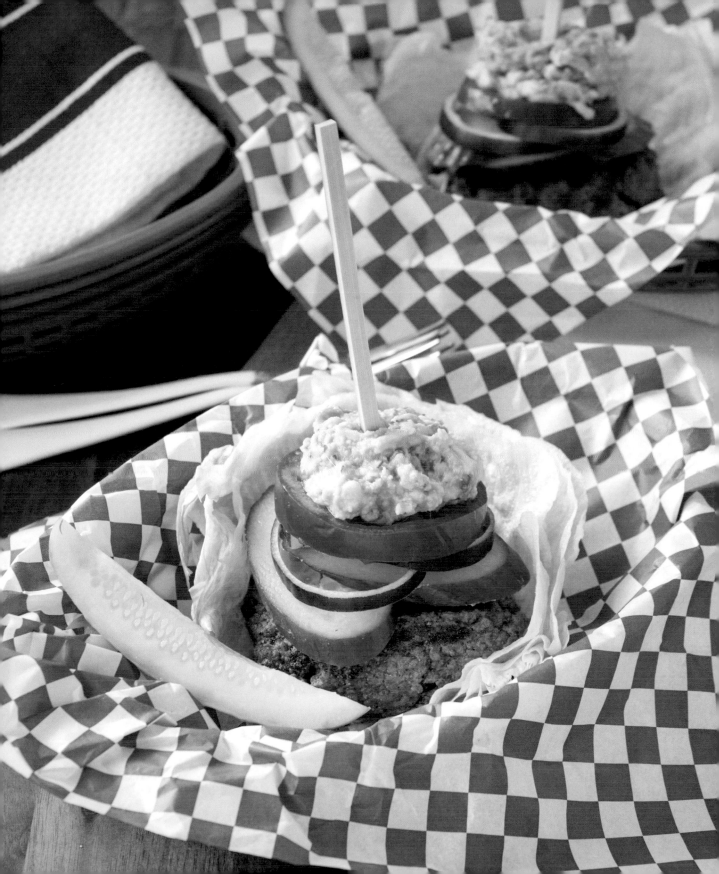

italian sausage & peppers

PREP TIME **10 MINS** • COOK TIME **30 MINS** • SERVINGS **4**

NUTS

EGGS

NIGHTSHADES

FODMAPS

SEAFOOD

1 pound ground pork

2 tablespoons Italian Sausage Spice Blend (page 222)

2 tablespoons coconut oil, divided

2 bell peppers, sliced

1/2 medium red onion, sliced

1/2 fennel bulb, sliced

1 tablespoon dried parsley

1 teaspoon granulated garlic

1 teaspoon onion powder

1 tablespoon dried basil

1/4 teaspoon dried thyme

1/4 teaspoon dried oregano

1/2 teaspoon sea salt

1 (14.5-ounce) can no-salt-added diced tomatoes

Roasted Garlic Parsnip Mash (page 148), for serving

Place the pork and Spice Blend in a medium bowl; mix together until thoroughly combined.

In a Dutch oven or high-sided saucepan over medium heat, melt 1 tablespoon of the coconut oil. Add the pork mixture to the pan and cook for about 10 minutes or until just a little pink is left. Remove the pork from the pan with a slotted spoon and set aside.

Place the remaining 1 tablespoon of coconut oil in the pan and add the bell peppers, onion, and fennel. Cook until the bell peppers start to soften, about 5 minutes. Sprinkle the parsley, granulated garlic, onion powder, basil, thyme, oregano, and salt over the peppers and stir for 30 seconds. Place the pork back in the pan and add the tomatoes; stir to mix well and reduce the heat to medium-low.

Simmer for 10 minutes or until sauce begins to thicken. Remove from the heat and let cool for 5 minutes before serving.

Serve over Roasted Garlic Parsnip Mash.

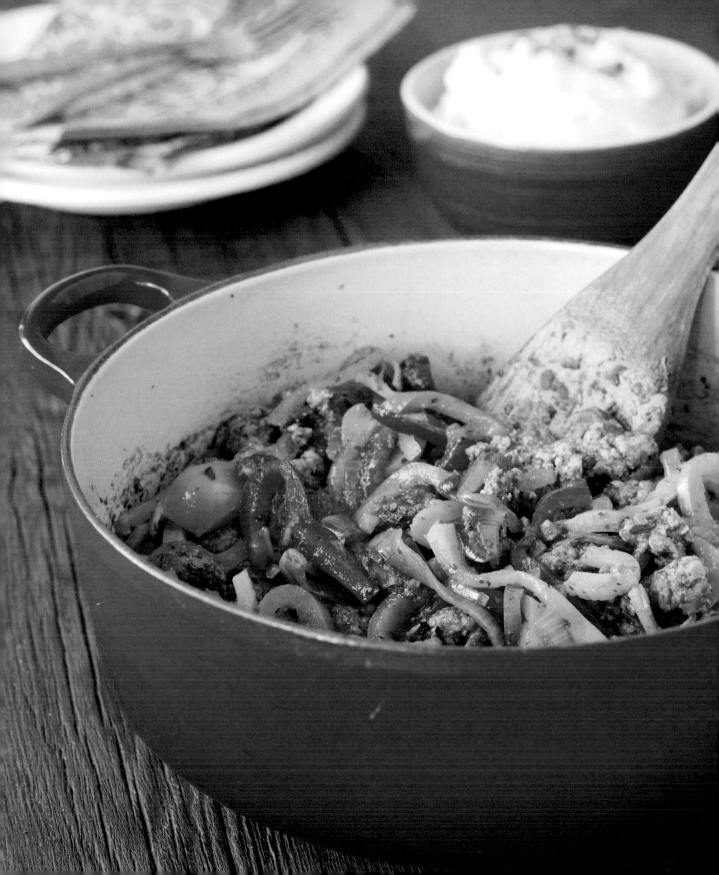

smoky grilled pork chops with cookout coleslaw

PREP TIME **15 MINS** • COOK TIME **15 MINS** • SERVINGS **4**

NUTS
EGGS
NIGHTSHADES
FODMAPS
SEAFOOD

1 tablespoon bacon fat or coconut oil

4 (1-inch-thick) bone-in pork chops (6 to 8 ounces each)

2 tablespoons Smoky Spice Blend (page 222)

FOR THE SLAW

3 tablespoons Healthy Homemade Mayonnaise (page 219)

3 tablespoons apple cider vinegar*

1 teaspoon gluten-free brown mustard*

1/2 teaspoon onion powder

1/2 teaspoon granulated garlic

1 teaspoon celery salt (or 1/2 teaspoon celery seed)

1/2 head green cabbage, finely sliced or shredded

1 large carrot, shredded

sea salt and black pepper to taste

Preheat the oven to 400°F.

Heat a grill or grill pan over medium-high heat, then brush with the bacon fat or coconut oil. Season the pork chops liberally on both sides with the Spice Blend, then place on the hot grill for 3 minutes per side. If using a grill pan, place the pan in the oven to continue cooking for 4 to 8 minutes or until the chops reach an internal temperature of 145°F. If you are grilling outside, move the chops to a higher rack or lower-temperature area of the grill to cook evenly until they've cooked through. Alternatively, you can transfer the chops from the grill to an oven-safe pan and finish cooking in the oven as described above.

Make the slaw: In a large mixing bowl, whisk together the Mayonnaise, vinegar, mustard, onion powder, granulated garlic, and celery salt. Add the cabbage and carrot and toss well to combine. Taste and add salt and pepper as desired. Note: When using celery salt, it's important to add it before you add sea salt to be sure you don't overseason the slaw.

Eat immediately, or refrigerate for several hours or overnight before serving. The slaw will soften over time.

INGREDIENT TIP
*Check out pages 226–227 for a list of recommended brands.

EGG FREE?
Make Spicy Slaw (page 134) instead of Cookout Coleslaw. ●

Make this with tuna steaks instead of pork chops and grill just 2 minutes per side.

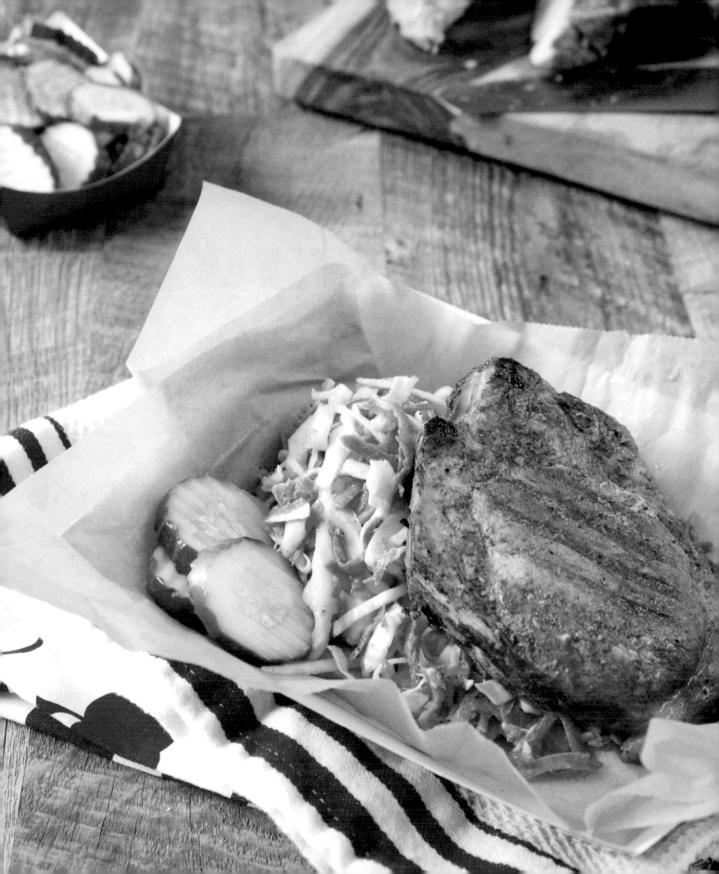

ahi tuna poke bowl

PREP TIME **20 MINS** • SERVINGS **4**

2 large cucumbers

sea salt and black pepper to taste

1 red bell pepper, thinly sliced

1 avocado, sliced

2 tablespoons coconut aminos*

juice of 1 lime

juice of 1/2 lemon

2 tablespoons organic rice vinegar

4 tablespoons cold-pressed sesame oil

1/4 cup sliced green onions (scallions)

1/4 cup finely diced red onion

pinch of red pepper flakes (optional)

1 to 1 1/2 pounds fresh, wild-caught, sushi-grade ahi tuna (or wild-caught salmon)

1/4 cup sliced nori* (optional)

2 tablespoons sesame seeds, divided

Cut the cucumbers into noodles using a handheld julienne peeler, a spiralizer tool, or even a regular vegetable peeler (if using a regular peeler, the noodles will be wide and flat instead of spaghetti-shaped). Season lightly with salt and pepper and portion into 4 serving bowls. Divide the bell pepper and avocado slices evenly among the bowls.

In a mixing bowl, whisk together the coconut aminos, lime and lemon juices, vinegar, and oil. Season with salt and pepper to taste. Add the green and red onions and red pepper flakes, if using.

Dice the tuna into 1/2-inch chunks as evenly as possible. Right before serving, toss the tuna with the sauce, nori, and 1 tablespoon of the sesame seeds. Portion the tuna evenly into the bowls. Garnish with the remaining sesame seeds.

Enjoy this dish by tossing everything together with chopsticks to mix the sauce throughout the ingredients.

INGREDIENT TIP
*Check out pages 226–227 for a list of recommended brands.

NIGHTSHADE FREE?
Omit the red bell pepper and use thinly sliced carrots instead. Omit the red pepper flakes

CHEF NOTE
The fish will turn whitish on the edges when tossed in the sauce. The acidity of the sauce, in effect, lightly "cooks" the fish, causing this change in appearance.

NO AHI? NO PROBLEM
You can easily make this dish using cooked strips of meat like skirt steak, chicken, or pork. ●

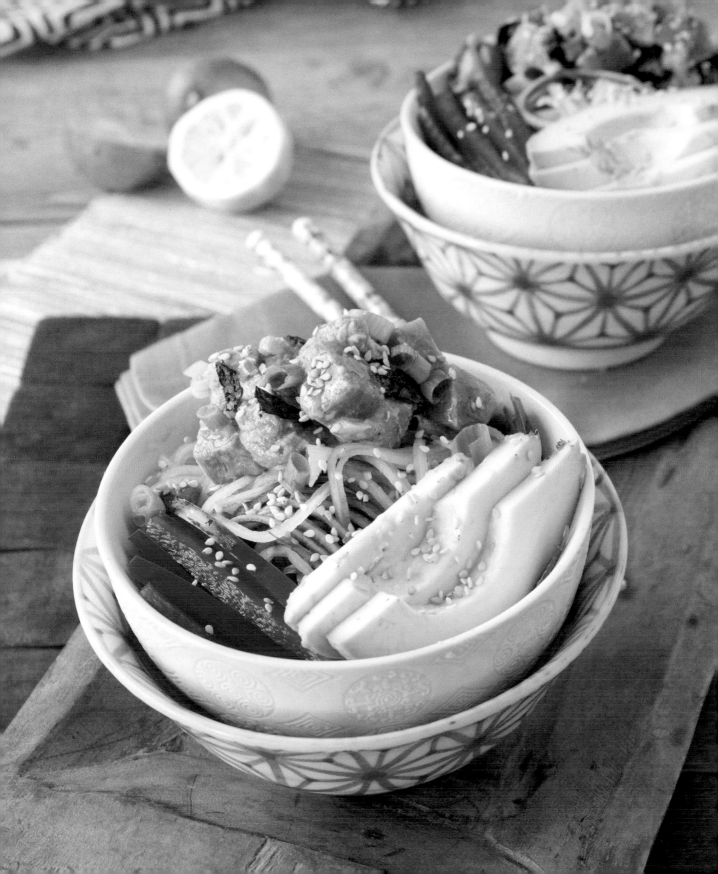

jalapeño-dill tuna salad

PREP TIME **10 MINS** • SERVINGS **4**

NUTS

EGGS

NIGHTSHADES

FODMAPS

SEAFOOD

3 (6-ounce) cans wild albacore tuna

2 jalapeño peppers, minced (remove ribs and seeds for less heat)

3 celery stalks, diced

1/2 cup diced red onion

1 recipe Healthy Homemade Mayonnaise (page 219)

3 tablespoons dried dill

1 1/2 teaspoons granulated garlic

sea salt and black pepper to taste

2 avocados, halved

lemon wedges for garnish

Drain the water or oil from the cans of tuna. Put the tuna in a medium bowl along with the jalapeños, celery, and onion and mix thoroughly.

In a small bowl, combine the Mayonnaise, dill, granulated garlic, salt, and pepper. Add the mayonnaise mixture to the tuna mixture and stir to combine.

Serve over the avocado halves with lemon wedges for garnish.

EGG FREE?
Omit the Mayonnaise and use 1/4 cup extra-virgin olive oil plus 2 tablespoons of lemon juice to dress the salad. ●

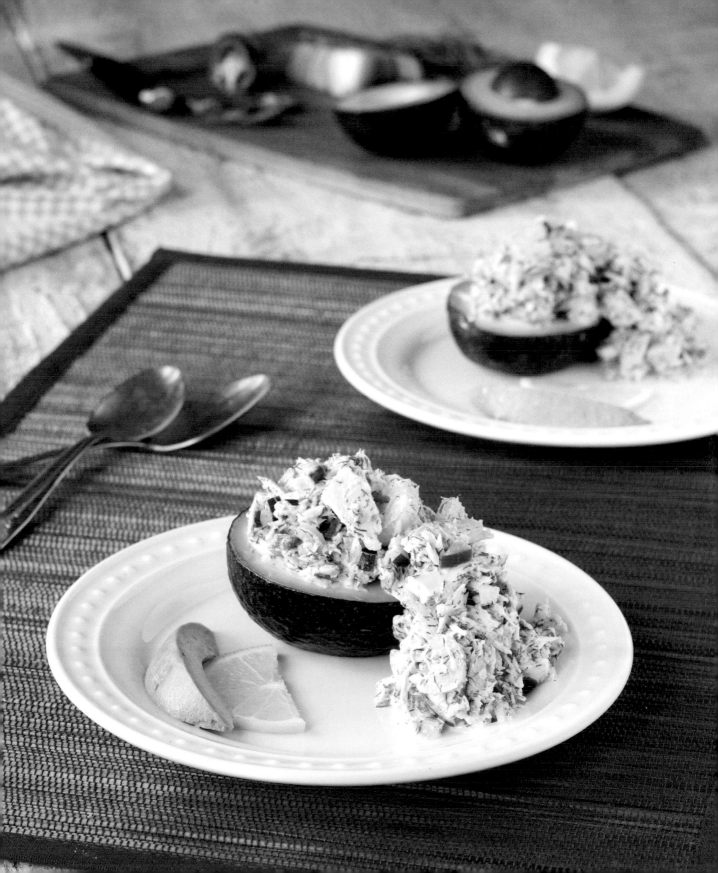

coconut-basil halibut with spinach

PREP TIME **15 MINS** • COOK TIME **15 TO 20 MINS** • SERVINGS **4**

NUTS

EGGS

NIGHTSHADES

FODMAPS

SEAFOOD

2 tablespoons coconut oil or ghee, divided

1/4 cup minced shallots

2 large cloves garlic, minced

3 teaspoons finely minced fresh ginger

1 small red chili pepper, thinly sliced

sea salt and black pepper

14.5 ounces full-fat coconut milk (about 1 3/4 cups), canned* or homemade (page 210)

juice of 1 lime

1/4 cup thinly sliced green onions (scallions)

3/4 cup fresh basil, sliced into a chiffonade (see Chef Note)

2 pounds halibut or other firm white fish fillets

6 cups spinach, packed

In a large skillet, melt 1 tablespoon of the coconut oil over medium heat. Add the shallots, garlic, ginger, and red chili and cook for 1 to 2 minutes or until the shallots and chilies start to soften. Season with salt and pepper. Pour in the coconut milk and lime juice and continue to cook for 2 to 3 minutes. Add the green onions and basil, giving it a quick stir to combine, and then place the fish fillets in the pan, spooning some of the coconut milk mixture over each fillet. Increase the heat to medium-high, and when the coconut milk mixture starts to bubble, turn the heat to low and cover the skillet. Cook for about 10 minutes or until the fish flakes easily with a fork.

While the fish is cooking, heat the remaining 1 tablespoon of coconut oil in another skillet over medium heat. Add the spinach, season with salt and pepper, and toss well to coat with the oil. Cook for 2 to 3 minutes or until the spinach is wilted.

To serve, divide the spinach among 4 serving plates or shallow bowls, top each with a piece of fish, and spoon some of the coconut milk mixture over the top.

INGREDIENT TIP
*Check out pages 226–227 for a list of recommended brands.

NIGHTSHADE FREE?
Omit the red chili pepper.

CHEF NOTE
To slice basil into a chiffonade, simply lay the leaves on top of one another, then roll them up together. Slice the rolled-up leaves crosswise to yield thin ribbons of basil. ●

Follow nightshade-free notes.

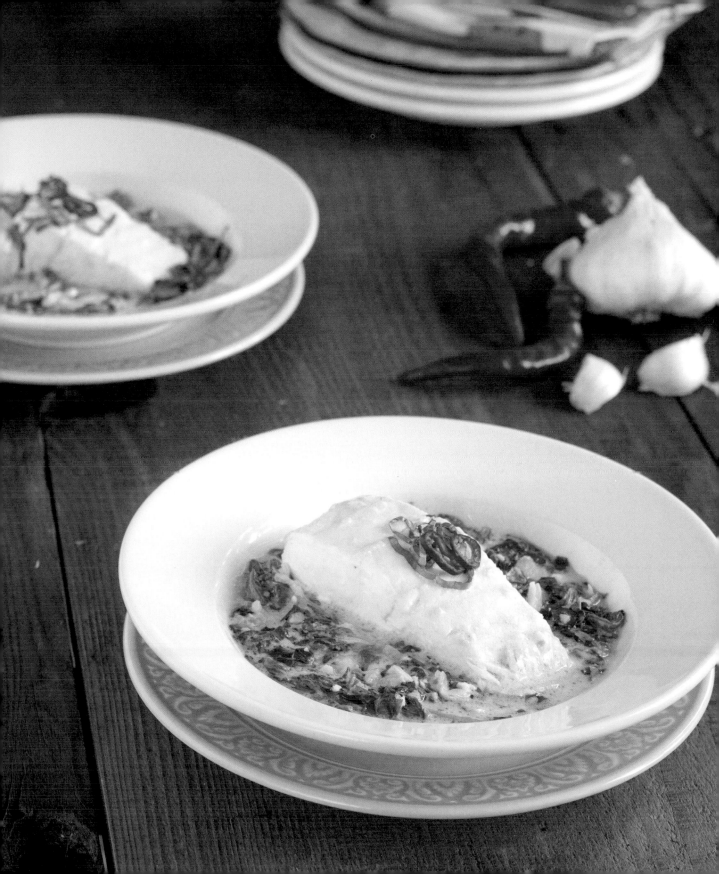

salmon with creamy tzatziki sauce & dill carrots

PREP TIME **15 MINS** • COOK TIME **10 TO 15 MINS** • SERVINGS **4**

NUTS

EGGS

NIGHTSHADES

FODMAPS

SEAFOOD

1/3 cup full-fat coconut milk, canned* or homemade (page 210)

1/2 cucumber, peeled and grated or shredded

1 small clove garlic, minced or grated

3 tablespoons chopped fresh dill, divided, plus 1 sprig for garnish

1 lemon, cut in half

sea salt and black pepper to taste

4 (6- to 8-ounce) wild-caught salmon fillets

3 tablespoons ghee or coconut oil, melted, divided

4 large carrots, cut into 1/4-by-3-inch sticks

INGREDIENT TIP
*Check out pages 226–227 for a list of recommended brands. ●

Place the oven rack in the top position and preheat the broiler to low.

Make the tzatziki sauce: In a small mixing bowl, combine the coconut milk, cucumber, garlic, 1 tablespoon of the chopped dill, and the juice of half of the lemon. Season with salt and pepper to taste.

Broil the salmon: Cut the remaining lemon half into thin slices. Place the salmon fillets in a broiler pan and brush them generously with 2 tablespoons of the ghee, then season liberally with salt and pepper. Top with the lemon slices and 1 tablespoon of the dill.

Broil for 8 to 12 minutes (depending on the thickness of the salmon), until it's cooked all the way through and turns from a darker to a lighter shade of pink. If you prefer slightly less well-done fish, broil for no more than 10 minutes.

Meanwhile, cook the carrots: In a large skillet over medium heat, melt the remaining 1 tablespoon of ghee, then place the carrots in the pan and season liberally with salt and pepper. Cover the pan and cook for 8 to 10 minutes or until the carrots are fork-tender. Add the remaining 1 tablespoon of dill to the pan and toss to combine.

Serve the salmon over the carrots and top with a generous drizzle of the tzatziki sauce. Garnish with a sprig of fresh dill.

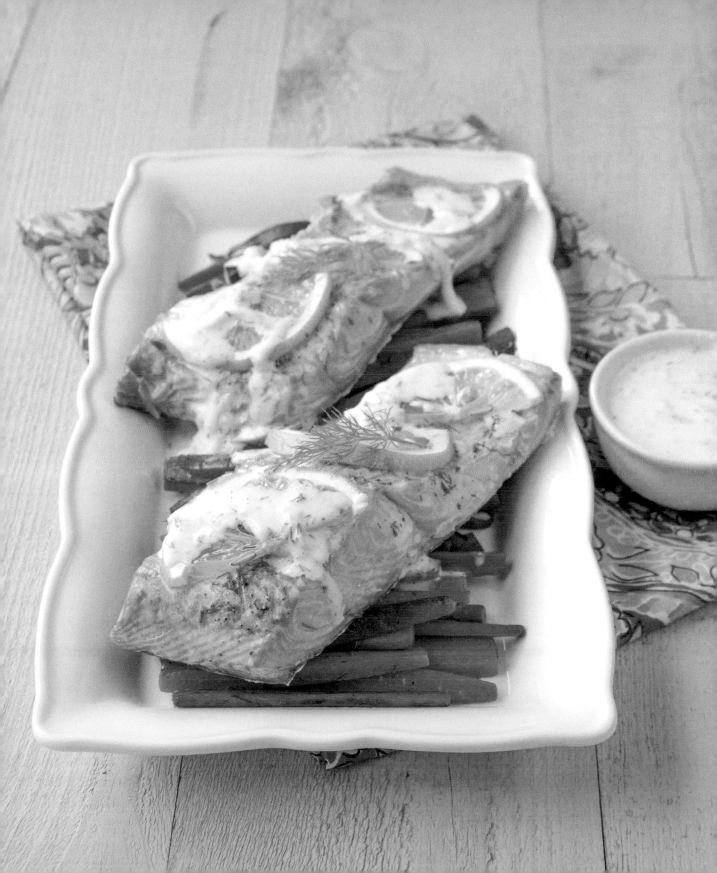

no-honey mustard pecan-crusted salmon

PREP TIME **10 MINS** • COOK TIME **15 MINS** • SERVINGS **4**

NUTS
EGGS
NIGHTSHADES
FODMAPS
SEAFOOD

1/2 cup finely chopped pecans

1/2 cup almond flour*

1 teaspoon sea salt, plus more for seasoning

1/4 cup finely chopped fresh parsley

4 (4- to 6-ounce) wild-caught salmon fillets

black pepper to taste

1/2 cup No-Honey Mustard Sauce (page 202), divided

Preheat the oven to 400°F. Line a rimmed baking sheet with parchment paper.

Combine the chopped pecans, almond flour, 1 teaspoon salt, and parsley in a small bowl.

Lay each salmon fillet, skin side down, on the prepared baking sheet and season with salt and pepper. Spread 2 tablespoons of the No-Honey Mustard Sauce on the top of each fillet. Put about 1/4 cup of the nut mixture on top of each fillet, gently pressing down. Bake the fillets for 12 to 15 minutes or until the thickest part of the fish flakes easily with a fork.

Serve with Caramelized Brussels Sprouts & Onions, page 150.

INGREDIENT TIP
*Check out pages 226–227 for a list of recommended brands. ●

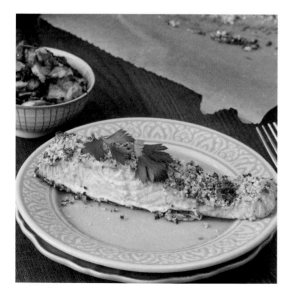

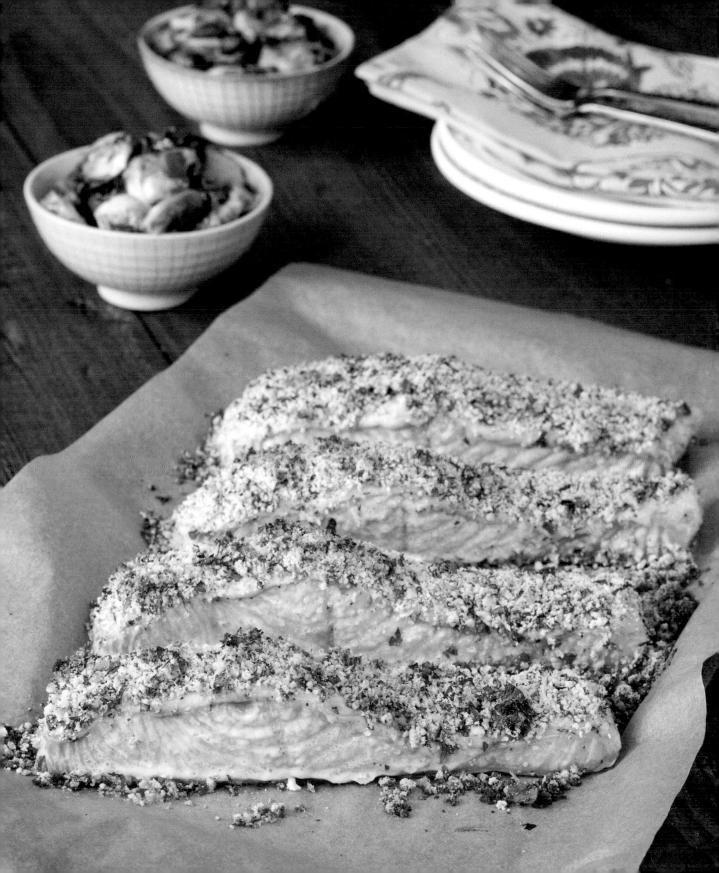

shrimp scampi with creamy garlic fettuccine

PREP TIME **20 MINS** • COOK TIME **15 MINS** • SERVINGS **4**

NUTS

EGGS

NIGHTSHADES

FODMAPS

SEAFOOD

4 tablespoons ghee, divided

2 teaspoons garlic, minced or grated

1 cup full-fat coconut milk, canned* or homemade (page 210)

sea salt and black pepper

4 large or 8 small zucchini

24 jumbo shrimp, peeled and deveined

INGREDIENT TIP
*Check out pages 226–227 for a list of recommended brands. ●

In a large, high-sided sauté pan or skillet over medium-low heat, melt 2 tablespoons of the ghee. Place the garlic in the pan and cook for 1 minute, allowing it to cook a bit but not to brown. Add the coconut milk to the pan and season generously with salt and pepper. Simmer the coconut milk until it is reduced by about half.

While the sauce simmers, use a vegetable peeler to turn the zucchini into fettuccine noodle–shaped strips by carefully "peeling" the entire length, down to the seeds; discard the seedy center. (I leave the skins on, but you can remove them first if you prefer.) Place the zucchini noodles in the reduced sauce and cook for about 5 minutes or until they're fork-tender and are cooked through to your liking. (Note that the zucchini will give off a good amount of water, so it's important to ensure that your coconut milk sauce is thick to maintain a less watery sauce.)

Plate the zucchini noodles, then increase the heat to medium. Add 1 tablespoon of ghee and 12 shrimp to the pan, season with salt and pepper, and cook for about 2 minutes per side or until the shrimp are pink and no longer translucent. Repeat this step for the remaining shrimp.

Serve the shrimp over the zucchini noodles. If you prefer to toss it all together, you may slice each piece of shrimp into 3 sections, removing the tail, and toss to combine with the zucchini.

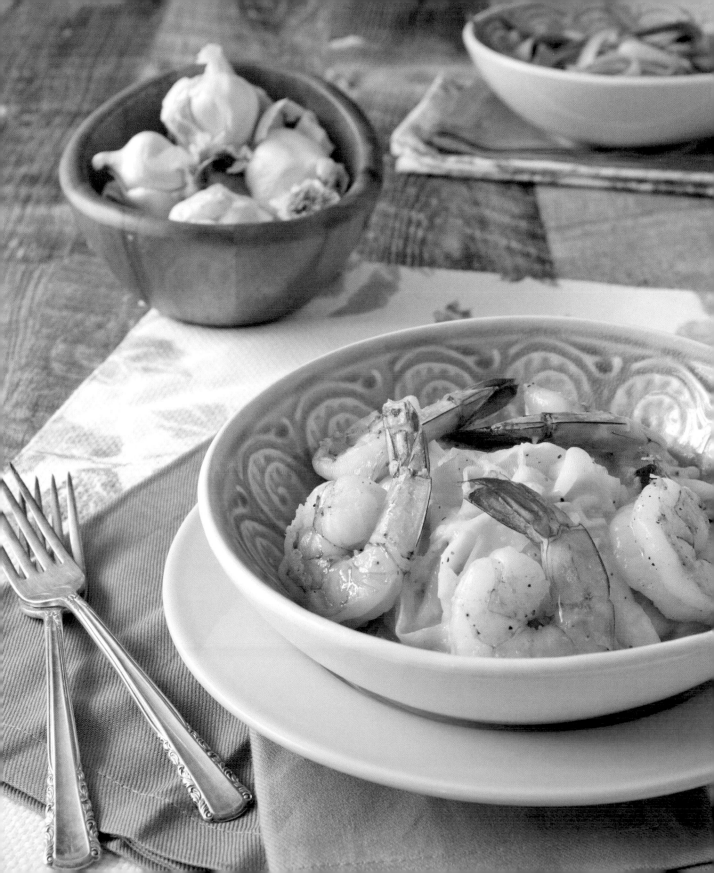

cabbage-wrapped dumplings

PREP TIME **30 MINS** • COOK TIME **20 MINS** • SERVINGS **4**

NUTS

EGGS

NIGHTSHADES

FODMAPS

SEAFOOD

INGREDIENT TIPS
*Refer to page 228 to see which fats are best for cooking.

**Check out pages 226–227 for a list of recommended brands.

SEAFOOD FREE?
Replace the shrimp with more pork.

DON'T EAT PORK?
Make these with just shrimp, or combine the shrimp with ground chicken or turkey instead of pork. ●

1 head napa cabbage, leaves separated and rinsed

FOR THE FILLING
2 cabbage leaves (from head of napa cabbage above)
1 tablespoon cooking fat*
1 celery stalk, minced (1/4 cup)
1/2 small onion, minced (1/4 cup)
1/2 small carrot, shredded (1/4 cup)
2 tablespoons coconut aminos**
3 drops fish sauce**
sea salt and black pepper
1/4 cup sliced green onions (scallions)
8 ounces shrimp, peeled and deveined, pulsed in food processor or minced
8 ounces ground pork
1/2 to 1 teaspoon minced fresh ginger
1 teaspoon minced garlic

FOR THE SAUCE
1/4 cup coconut aminos**
2 tablespoons cold-pressed sesame oil
2 teaspoons organic rice vinegar
3 drops fish sauce**
1 tablespoon fresh lime juice
2 tablespoons sliced green onions (scallions)

Place all but 2 of the large cabbage leaves in a large steamer basket over 1 inch of boiling water. Steam for 5 minutes or until the leaves become brighter green and pliable, then set them aside until the filling is cooked.

Make the filling: Slice the remaining raw cabbage leaves into very thin strips. In a large skillet over medium heat, melt the cooking fat and then sauté the celery, onion, carrot, and cabbage strips together with the coconut aminos and fish sauce. Season with salt and pepper to taste. When the vegetables are soft, about 5 minutes, add the green onions, shrimp, ground pork, ginger, and garlic to the pan. Stir well to combine, breaking up the pieces of meat so that the meat and vegetables are evenly dispersed. Once the pork is no longer pink and the shrimp is no longer translucent, about 5 minutes, remove the mixture from the heat.

Lay a cabbage leaf on a flat surface and spoon about 2 tablespoons of the filling into the center. Fold the end up around the filling, then the sides, and continue to roll the dumpling until it is wrapped. Secure the end of the cabbage leaf with a toothpick so that it remains tightly wrapped against the dumpling, holding the filling inside. Continue with the remaining cabbage leaves and filling until all the ingredients are used up.

Make the sauce: Whisk together all the sauce ingredients in a small mixing bowl.

Serve the dumplings warm with the sauce on the side for dipping.

 Make this with double the shrimp and omit the pork.

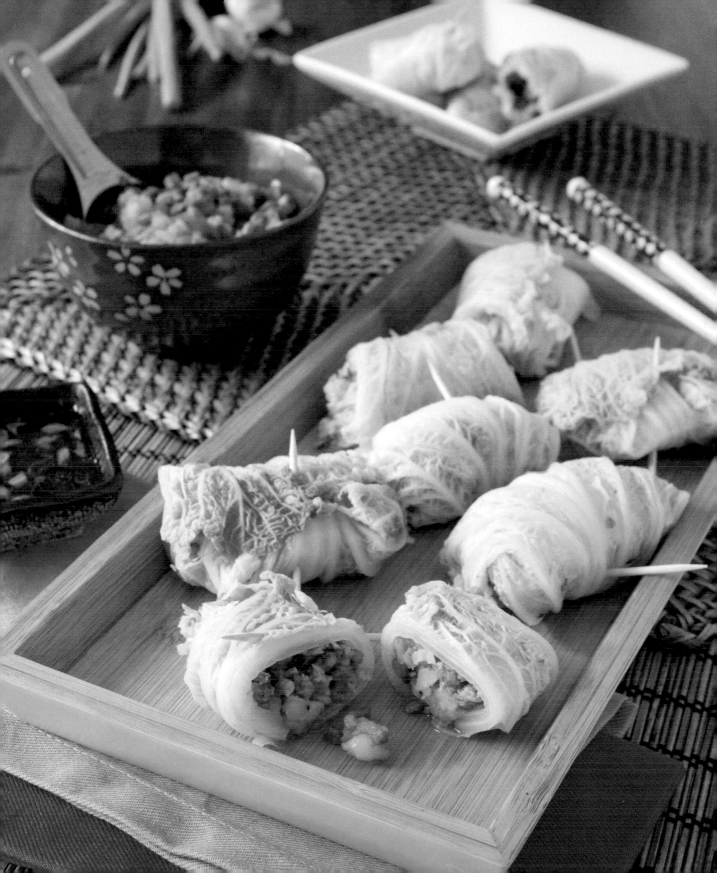

cilantro shrimp stir-fry

PREP TIME **10 MINS** • COOK TIME **10 TO 15 MINS** • SERVINGS **4**

NUTS

EGGS

NIGHTSHADES

FODMAPS

SEAFOOD

4 tablespoons ghee or coconut oil, divided

1 large red onion, sliced (1 cup)

sea salt and black pepper

1 large bell pepper, sliced (1 cup)

1 dozen small mushrooms, sliced (1 cup)

2 medium zucchini, sliced (1 cup)

3 to 4 cloves garlic, minced

1/2 teaspoon minced fresh ginger

3/4 cup minced fresh cilantro

2 dozen jumbo shrimp, peeled and deveined (and defrosted if frozen)

1 to 2 teaspoons ground coriander

1 lime, cut into wedges, for serving

In a large skillet or wok over medium-high heat, melt 2 tablespoons of the ghee, then add the onion and season generously with salt and pepper. Allow the onion slices to cook until they are translucent and the edges start to brown, about 3 to 4 minutes. Add the bell pepper, mushrooms, zucchini, garlic, and ginger and stir to combine and distribute the garlic and ginger throughout the pan. Season again with salt and pepper, add the cilantro, stir to incorporate, and cook the vegetables until tender, 3 to 5 minutes.

On a large plate, season the shrimp lightly on both sides with salt, pepper, and the coriander. When the vegetables are cooked, remove them from the pan and set aside. Reduce the heat to medium and add the remaining 2 tablespoons of ghee to the pan. Place the shrimp in the pan and cook for 2 minutes per side or until they're pink on the outside and opaque (no longer translucent) all the way through.

Serve the vegetables topped with 6 shrimp per person. Garnish with a lime wedge to squeeze over the dish before eating.

NIGHTSHADE-FREE?
Omit the bell pepper and bump up the other veggies.

KITCHEN TIP
This dish is perfect served over Garlic & Green Onion Cauli-Rice, page 136. ●

Follow nightshade-free notes.

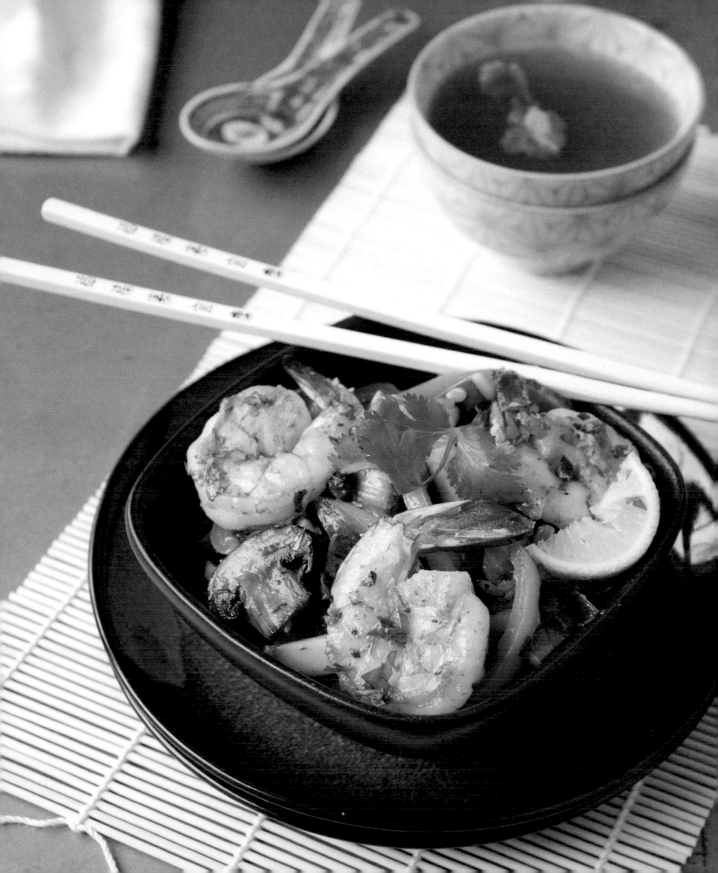

vegetable lasagne

PREP TIME **20 MINS** • COOK TIME **60 MINS** • SERVINGS **4**

NUTS

EGGS

NIGHTSHADES

FODMAPS

SEAFOOD

FOR THE SAUCE

1 tablespoon ghee or other cooking fat*

1 small yellow onion, diced

2 cloves garlic, minced

1 (14.5-ounce) can diced tomatoes**

6 large fresh basil leaves, sliced, plus extra leaves for optional garnish

sea salt and black pepper

FOR THE VEGETABLES

1 large eggplant

3 tablespoons ghee or other cooking fat*, divided, plus more for greasing the pan

sea salt and black pepper

1 dozen cremini or white button mushrooms, sliced

2 tablespoons water

1/2 pound baby spinach (about 4 cups)

1/2 teaspoon granulated garlic

INGREDIENT TIP

*Refer to page 228 to see which fats are best for cooking.

**Check out pages 226–227 for a list of recommended brands

CHEF NOTE

Try spreading some of the Herb Almond "Cheese" Spread (page 170) on top of each layer eggplant in the lasagne for added texture and flavor. ●

Preheat the oven to 350°F.

Prepare the sauce (this can be done ahead of time): In a saucepan over medium heat, melt the ghee. Add the onion and cook until it becomes translucent, about 3 to 5 minutes. Add the garlic and cook for 1 more minute, then add the tomatoes, basil, and a dash of salt and pepper. Reduce the heat to medium-low and simmer for 10 minutes. Taste for seasoning and add more salt and pepper if needed.

Prepare the vegetables: Slice the eggplant lengthwise into 1/4-inch-thick planks and place on rimmed baking sheet lined with parchment paper. Brush with 2 tablespoons of the ghee and season liberally with salt and pepper. Bake for 15 minutes.

In a large skillet over medium heat, melt the remaining 1 tablespoon of ghee. Add the mushrooms and cook until they are browned and softened, about 8 minutes. Remove the mushrooms from the pan and place them on a paper towel to drain. Add the water to the pan and then add the spinach and garlic. Cover and allow the spinach to wilt, about 2 to 3 minutes. Set the cooked spinach on a paper towel or in a colander to drain.

Assemble the lasagne: Grease a 9-by-13-inch baking dish with ghee, then begin to layer the vegetables and sauce, starting with the strips of eggplant, topping with a thin layer of sauce, then the spinach. Next, layer more eggplant, then sauce, then mushrooms. Repeat until all of the ingredients are used up, reserving some sauce and vegetables for the top layer.

Bake the lasagne for 30 minutes or until bubbling around the edges. Garnish with whole fresh basil leaves, if desired.

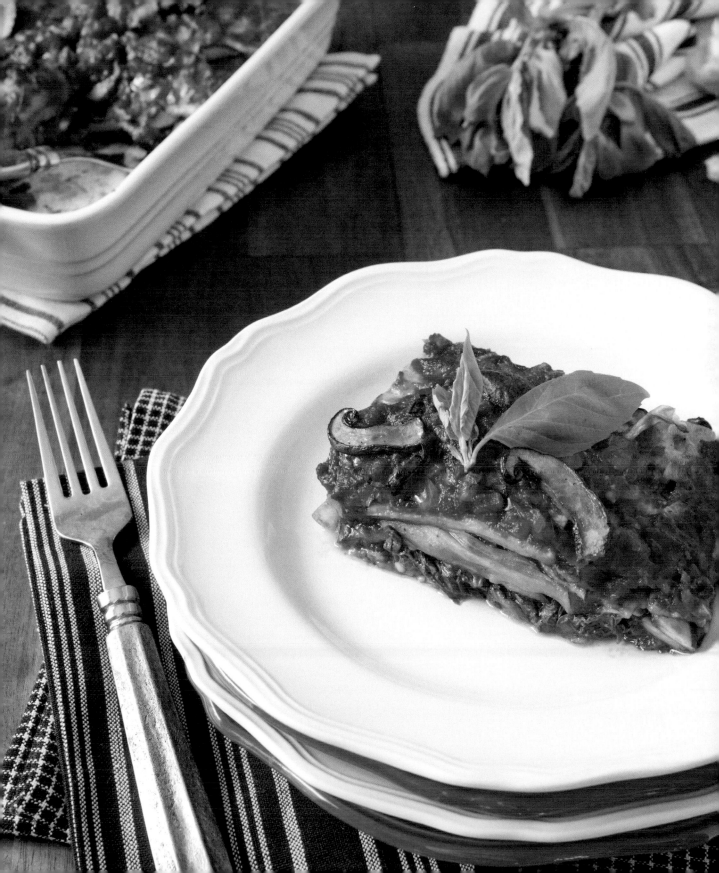

carrot-ginger soup

PREP TIME **10 MINS (+BROTH PREP)** • COOK TIME **15 TO 20 MINS** • SERVINGS **4**

NUTS

EGGS

NIGHTSHADES

FODMAPS

SEAFOOD

1 tablespoon ghee or other cooking fat*

1 celery stalk, diced (1/2 cup)

1/2 small yellow onion, diced (1/2 cup)

sea salt and black pepper

1 teaspoon minced garlic

1/2 to 1 teaspoon minced fresh ginger

6 extra-large carrots, chopped (4 cups)

3 cups Bone Broth, chicken (page 208), or Vegetable Broth (page 208)

a few sprigs fresh dill, for garnish (optional)

In a large pot over medium heat, melt the ghee. Cook the celery and onion with a dash of salt and pepper until they become tender and translucent, about 5 minutes. Stir in the garlic and ginger and cook for 1 minute, being careful not to burn the garlic. Add the carrots and Bone Broth, reduce the heat to medium-low, and simmer until the carrots are soft all the way through, about 10 minutes.

Transfer to a blender in 3 small batches, removing the center "valve" from the lid and covering the hole where the valve normally rests with a thick kitchen towel. Holding the lid in place with your hand, blend on low, then move to high speed after a few seconds. Note that blending hot liquids causes them to expand, so rushing to blend this all at once or in an overfilled blender is not safe and will cause hot soup to splatter everywhere. After blending all 3 batches, serve with a garnish of fresh dill, if using.

INGREDIENT TIP
*Refer to page 228 to see which fats are best for cooking.

KITCHEN TIP
You can make this soup a lot faster by steaming the diced carrots the day before or in a separate pot so that you don't need to wait for them to cook in the liquid with the soup. This will shave about 10 minutes off of your cooking time. ●

 Use sweet potatoes instead of carrots and simmer for 20 minutes instead of 10 to cook through.

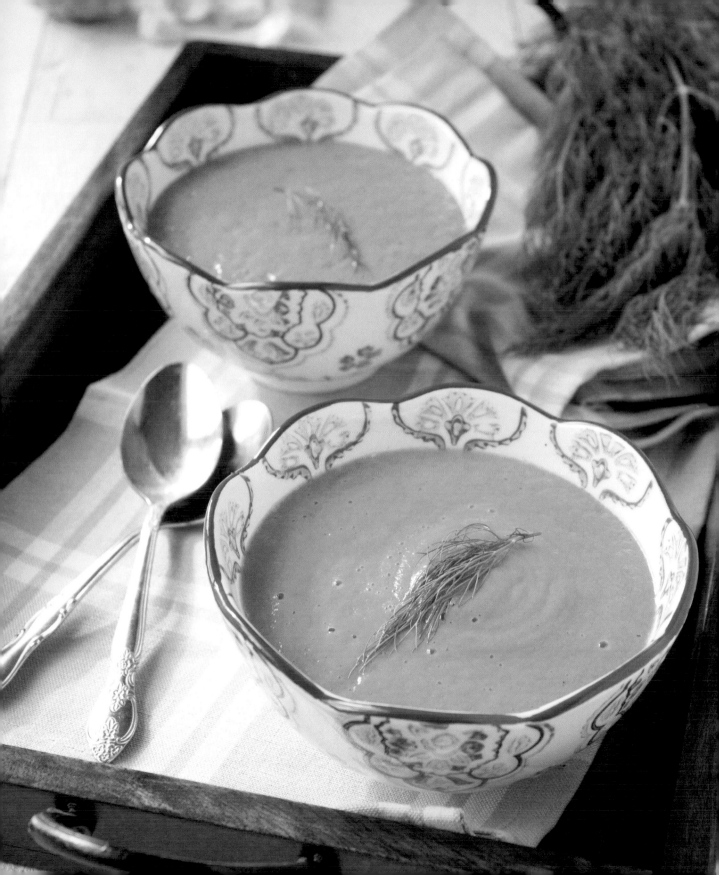

roasted cauliflower-leek soup

PREP TIME **15 MINS** • COOK TIME **35 MINS** • SERVINGS **4** • YIELD **4 CUPS**

NUTS

EGGS

NIGHTSHADES

FODMAPS

SEAFOOD

1 head cauliflower, coarsely chopped (2 to 3 cups)

2 leeks, sliced into 1/2-inch lengths (white and very light green portions only)

6 cloves garlic

2 tablespoons coconut oil, melted

1 1/2 cups Bone Broth, chicken (page 208), or Vegetable Broth (page 208)

1 teaspoon sea salt

1/4 teaspoon white pepper

1/4 cup full-fat coconut milk, canned* or homemade (page 210)

1 teaspoon red pepper flakes (optional)

a few thinly sliced leeks, for garnish (optional)

Celery Root Cakes (page 168), for serving (optional)

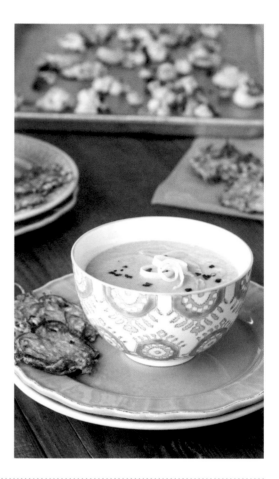

INGREDIENT TIP
*Check out pages 226–227 for a list of recommended brands.

CHEF NOTE
Use the Vegetable Broth to make this recipe pescetarian-friendly.

NIGHTSHADE FREE?
Don't add the red pepper flakes. ●

Follow nightshade-free notes.

Preheat the oven to 400°F. On 2 large rimmed baking sheets, spread out the cauliflower, leeks, and garlic cloves in a single layer. Drizzle with the coconut oil and toss to fully coat each piece. Place in the oven and roast for 25 to 35 minutes, rotating the pans halfway through. When you rotate the pans, check the leeks and pull them out if they start to brown more quickly.

Place the roasted cauliflower, leeks, and garlic in a blender with the Bone Broth and purée for about 3 minutes or until the mixture is smooth. Add the salt, pepper, coconut milk, and red pepper flakes, if using, and blend for 20 to 30 seconds or until well incorporated.

When you're ready to serve, bring the mixture to a simmer in a saucepan over low heat. Garnish with thinly sliced leeks and red pepper flakes.

This soup pairs perfectly with the Celery Root Cakes.

weeknight chicken soup

PREP TIME **10 MINS** • COOK TIME **30 TO 35 MINS** • SERVINGS **4**

NUTS

EGGS

NIGHTSHADES

FODMAPS

SEAFOOD

1 pound boneless, skinless chicken thighs

sea salt and black pepper

2 tablespoons cooking fat*

1 small onion, diced (3/4 cup)

2 large celery stalks, diced (3/4 cup)

1 extra-large or 2 medium carrots, diced (3/4 cup)

4 cups Bone Broth, chicken (page 208)

2 tablespoons chopped fresh dill, plus more for garnish

INGREDIENT TIP
*Refer to page 228 to see which fats are best for cooking.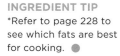

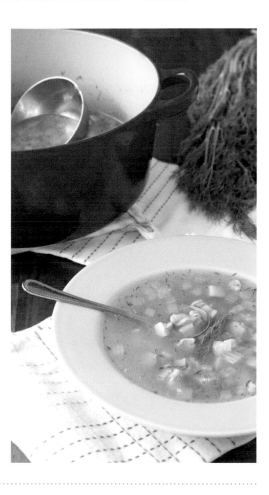

Preheat oven to 350°F.

Season the chicken thighs liberally with salt and pepper. Place them on a rimmed baking sheet pan and bake for 30 to 35 minutes or until the internal temperature of the chicken reaches 165°F. When the chicken is finished cooking, chop it into small chunks.

In a large pot over medium heat, melt the cooking fat. Add the onion, celery, and carrots, season with salt and pepper, and sauté for 5 to 8 minutes or until the vegetables are fork-tender and the onions are translucent.

Add the Bone Broth and chunks of chicken to the pot and simmer for 10 minutes to marry the flavors. Stir in the dill just before serving and garnish with more dill if you like.

This soup pairs perfectly with the Dill Crackers on page 163.

portuguese green soup
(caldo verde)

PREP TIME **20 MINS** • COOK TIME **30 MINS** • SERVINGS **4**

NUTS

EGGS

NIGHTSHADES

FODMAPS

SEAFOOD

1 pound ground pork

3 tablespoons Chorizo
Spice Blend (page 222)

2 tablespoons coconut oil

1/2 medium yellow onion,
diced

3 cloves garlic, minced

4 cups Bone Broth,
chicken (page 208)

4 cups water

3 large parsnips, peeled
and sliced very thin

1 teaspoon sea salt

1/2 teaspoon black pepper

1 bunch of kale, any kind
(1 pound)

In a medium bowl, thoroughly combine the ground pork and Spice Blend.

In a large pot over medium heat, crumble the chorizo-spiced pork into large pieces and cook until almost no pink remains, about 10 minutes. Remove the pork from the pan with a slotted spoon and set aside in a small bowl.

In the same pot, over medium-high heat, add the coconut oil, onion, and garlic and sauté until the onion just becomes translucent, 2 to 3 minutes. Add the Bone Broth, water, parsnips, salt, and pepper to the pot and bring to a boil. Reduce the heat to medium, cover, and cook until the parsnips are fork-tender, about 15 minutes.

While the parsnips are cooking, remove the stems and thick middle rib from each kale leaf and form stacks of 4 to 5 leaves. From one side of each stack of leaves to the other, roll up the leaves into a tight roll. Starting from one end of the roll, use a knife to cut the kale into 1/4-inch strips. Continue this process until all the kale is sliced.

Once the parsnips are soft, use an immersion blender or potato masher to blend or mash the parsnips in the pot. Add the cooked pork and the sliced kale and cook until the kale is softened, about 5 minutes. Season with additional salt and pepper to taste.

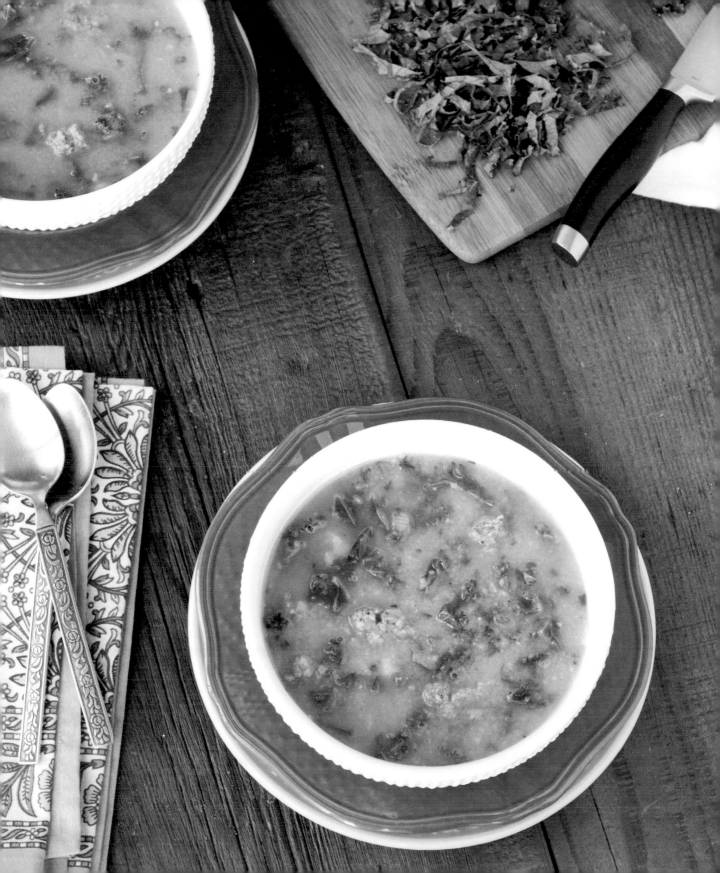

creamy mushroom soup

PREP TIME **10 MINS** • COOK TIME **20 MINS** • SERVINGS **4**

NUTS

EGGS

NIGHTSHADES

FODMAPS

SEAFOOD

1 tablespoon bacon fat or ghee

1/2 medium onion, diced (1 cup)

sea salt and black pepper

1 dozen medium-sized mushrooms (cremini or shiitake), sliced

leaves from 1 sprig fresh thyme (1/2 teaspoon), plus an additional sprig for optional garnish

pinch of nutmeg

3 1/2 cups Bone Broth, beef (page 208)

1/2 cup full-fat coconut milk, canned* or homemade (page 210)

In a large saucepan or soup pot, melt the bacon fat over medium heat, then cook the onion until it is translucent and the edges begin to brown, about 5 minutes. Season lightly with salt and pepper.

Add the mushrooms, thyme leaves, and nutmeg to the pan. Continue to cook until the mushrooms brown, about 10 minutes.

Add the Bone Broth and coconut milk and simmer for 5 minutes.

Using a slotted spoon, remove 1/2 cup of the mushrooms from the pan and set aside. (For a completely creamy soup without any chunks of mushroom, skip this step.)

Transfer the soup to a blender in 3 small batches, removing the center "valve" from the lid and covering the hole where the valve normally rests with a thick kitchen towel. Holding the lid in place with your hand, blend on low, then move to high speed after a few seconds. Note that blending hot liquids causes them to expand, so rushing to blend this all at once or in an overfilled blender is not safe and will cause hot soup to splatter everywhere.

After blending all 3 batches, pour the soup into serving bowls and evenly distribute the reserved mushrooms. Garnish with a portion of a thyme sprig, if desired.

INGREDIENT TIP
*Check out pages 226–227 for a list of recommended brands.

DON'T EAT BEEF?
Use Vegetable Broth (page 208) instead of Beef Broth. ●

Make this with Vegetable Broth (page 208) instead of beef.

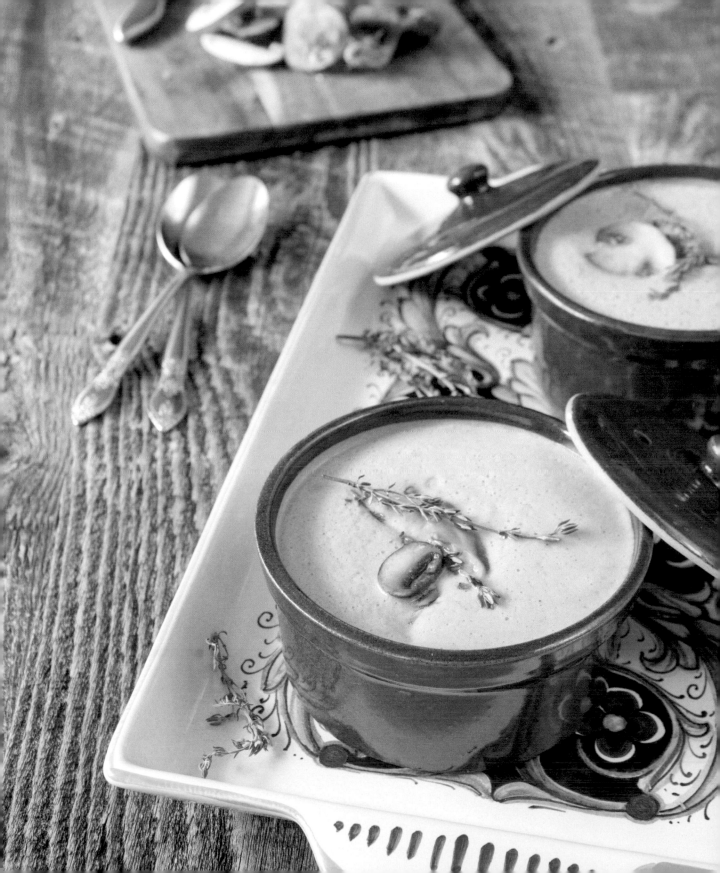

NUTS

EGGS

NIGHTSHADES

FODMAPS

SEAFOOD

spicy slaw

PREP TIME **20 MINS** • YIELD **5 CUPS**

1/4 cup nut or seed butter (almond, walnut, or sesame tahini or Sunbutter, page 164)

juice of 1 lime

4 cloves garlic, minced

1 to 2 tablespoons Garlic Chili Paste (page 196), depending on desired heat level

2 teaspoons fish sauce,* or more to taste

4 cups cabbage, finely shredded (1 medium head)

2 large carrots, finely shredded

4 green onions (scallions), sliced

1/2 cup diced red onion

1 to 2 jalapeño peppers, thinly sliced (optional)

INGREDIENT TIP
*Check out pages 226–227 for a list of recommended brands.

NIGHTSHADE FREE?
Omit the jalapeños. ●

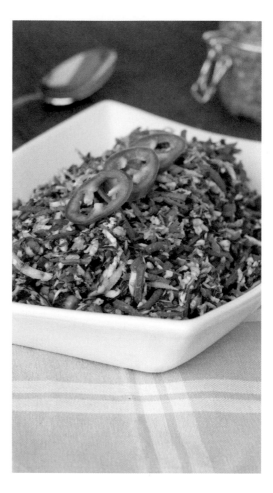

Combine the nut or seed butter, lime juice, garlic, Garlic Chili Paste, and fish sauce in a small bowl and whisk until combined.

Place the cabbage, carrots, green onions, red onion, and jalapeños, if using, in a large bowl and toss until the ingredients are evenly distributed. Pour the nut butter mixture over the cabbage mixture and combine thoroughly. For better flavor, refrigerate for at least an hour before serving.

beet & carrot stacked salad

PREP TIME **15 MINS** • SERVINGS **4**

SOUPS
SALADS
& SIDES

FOR THE DRESSING

juice of 2 lemons

1/4 cup extra-virgin olive oil

1/4 cup chopped fresh cilantro or basil, plus more for garnish

sea salt and black pepper to taste

1 green apple

1 large cucumber

1 medium beet, peeled and shredded (1 cup)

2 large carrots, shredded (1 cup)

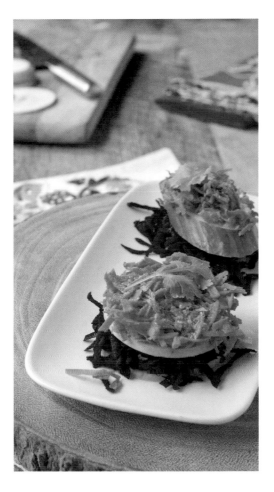

NUTS

EGGS

NIGHTSHADES

FODMAPS

SEAFOOD

CHEF NOTE
Another way to make this salad is to simply shred both the apple and the cucumber along with the carrots and beets, then toss all the shredded vegetables and fruit together with the dressing to make a tasty slaw. ●

Make the dressing: Combine all the dressing ingredients in a small mixing bowl.

Assemble the salads: Slice the green apple thinly into 8 discs, 1/4-inch or thinner. Slice the cucumber on the bias to create 8 ovals with a greater surface area than if you had sliced directly across to make rounds.

On a salad plate, place 2 tablespoons of the shredded beets on top of an apple slice and cover with 1 tablespoon of the dressing. Stack another apple slice on top of the beets, then 2 tablespoons of the carrots and another 1 tablespoon of the dressing. Repeat this process using all of the apple and cucumber slices to make a total of 8 stacks. Serve each person 2 stacks—1 each of apple and cucumber.

garlic & green onion cauli-rice

PREP TIME **10 MINS** • COOK TIME **10 MINS** • SERVINGS **4**

1 large head cauliflower

2 tablespoons ghee or coconut oil

3 cloves garlic, minced

3 green onions (scallions), thinly sliced

sea salt and black pepper to taste

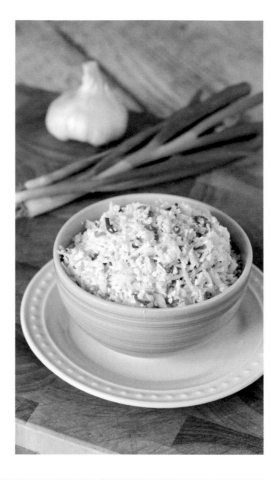

Shred the cauliflower with a cheese grater or food processor. Heat the ghee in a large sauté pan over medium-high heat. Add the garlic and sauté for 2 to 3 minutes or until fragrant. Add the green onions and cook for another 1 to 2 minutes, then add the shredded cauliflower and stir to combine with the garlic and green onion. Cook for 3 to 5 minutes or until the dish is warmed through and the cauliflower is softened. Season with salt and pepper to taste.

moroccan cauli-rice pilaf

PREP TIME **20 MINS** • COOK TIME **15 MINS** • SERVINGS **4**

NUTS

EGGS

NIGHTSHADES

FODMAPS

SEAFOOD

3 tablespoons ghee or
   coconut oil

1 medium yellow onion, diced

3 cloves garlic, minced

1 teaspoon sea salt

1/2 teaspoon ground ginger

1/4 teaspoon white pepper

1 teaspoon ground cumin

1 teaspoon ground turmeric

1 large head cauliflower,
   shredded

1/2 cup fresh cilantro,
   chopped, plus more for
   optional garnish

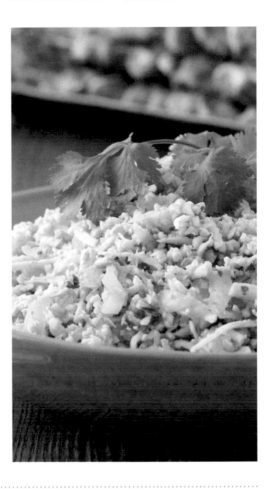

Heat the ghee in a deep skillet over medium-high heat. Add the onion and garlic and sauté for 3 to 5 minutes or until the onion is translucent. Sprinkle the salt, ginger, white pepper, cumin, and turmeric over the onion-garlic mixture and stir for about 30 seconds or until fragrant. Add the shredded cauliflower and cilantro and mix until the color of the seasonings is well dispersed. Reduce the heat to low, cover, and cook for 3 to 5 minutes or until the cauliflower is tender. Garnish with 1 or 2 stems of fresh cilantro, if desired.

brussels sprouts with
crispy capers & bacon

PREP TIME **15 MINS** • COOK TIME **40 MINS** • SERVINGS **4**

NUTS

EGGS

NIGHTSHADES

FODMAPS

SEAFOOD

4 slices bacon

2 dozen Brussels sprouts

sea salt and black pepper

coconut oil for frying the capers

1/4 cup capers, drained

zest of 1 lemon

juice of 1/2 lemon

Preheat the oven to 350°F.

In a large, deep pot over medium-low heat, cook the bacon for about 8 minutes or until the fat has rendered off and the bacon is crispy. Remove the bacon from the pot and pour the bacon grease onto a large rimmed baking sheet.

Slice the bottoms off of the Brussels sprouts, then quarter them. Place them on the baking sheet and toss to coat evenly with the bacon grease. Season lightly with salt and pepper. Roast the Brussels sprouts for approximately 30 minutes or until the edges begin to brown and they become bright green.

While the Brussels sprouts roast, add about 1/4 inch of coconut oil to the pot used to cook the bacon. Once the oil is hot, carefully place the capers in the oil and cover with a splatter screen, as a lot of water in the capers will cook off and splatter in the first few seconds. Fry the capers for 1 to 2 minutes or until they become darker green and crispy. Set them aside.

When the Brussels sprouts are finished roasting, chop the bacon into 1/4-inch pieces and sprinkle it over the top along with the capers and lemon zest. Pour the lemon juice over the top and serve warm.

KITCHEN TIP

A large, deep pot is useful in this case because dropping capers, which have a fair amount of water in them, into hot oil will cause splattering. The depth of the pot helps to contain the splattering that naturally occurs in this process. ●

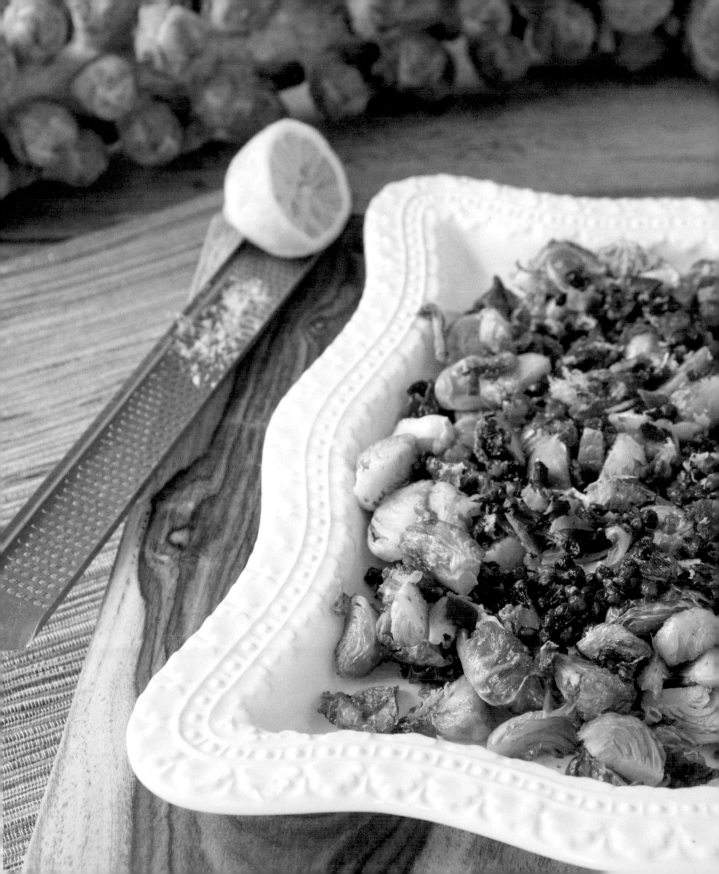

NUTS

EGGS

NIGHTSHADES

FODMAPS

SEAFOOD

asian sautéed greens

PREP TIME **5 MINS** • COOK TIME **5 MINS** • SERVINGS **4**

1 head bok choy (or 8 baby bok choy)

2 tablespoons coconut oil or other cooking fat*

1/4 cup coconut aminos**

4 drops fish sauce**

1/2 teaspoon minced or grated garlic

2 teaspoons cold-pressed sesame oil, to finish

2 teaspoons sesame seeds, for garnish

INGREDIENT TIPS

*Refer to page 228 to see which fats are best for cooking.

**Check out pages 226–227 for a list of recommended brands.

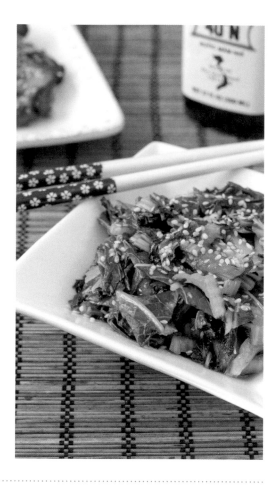

Slice the green leafy portion of the bok choy crosswise into 1-inch strips and the mostly white portion into 1/4-inch strips—this will allow all the parts to cook evenly. Discard the very end of the bulb.

In a large, high-sided sauté pan or skillet over medium-high heat, melt the coconut oil, then add the bok choy, coconut aminos, fish sauce, and garlic. Cook, covered, for 2 minutes, then reduce the heat and cook, uncovered, for an additional 2 to 3 minutes or until the greens are completely wilted and softened and some of the water cooks off of the greens.

Serve warm, garnished with sesame oil and sesame seeds.

This dish pairs perfectly with the Lemon Ginger Chicken on page 72 or the Asian Ginger Flank Steak on page 88.

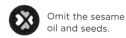
Omit the sesame oil and seeds.

braised balsamic red cabbage

PREP TIME **10 MINS** • COOK TIME **25 TO 30 MINS** • SERVINGS **4**

2 tablespoons coconut oil

1 medium yellow onion, sliced

sea salt and black pepper

1 medium cabbage, cored and sliced

1/4 cup Bone Broth, beef or chicken (page 208), or Vegetable Broth (208)

2 tablespoons balsamic vinegar or apple cider vinegar*

1/2 teaspoon dried rosemary, finely chopped

NUTS

EGGS

NIGHTSHADES

FODMAPS

SEAFOOD

INGREDIENT TIP
*Check out pages 226–227 for a list of recommended brands. ●

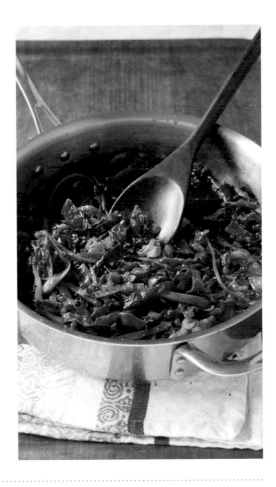

In a large stainless-steel sauté pan or enameled pot, melt the coconut oil over medium heat. Add the onion to the pan and season lightly with salt and pepper. After about 5 minutes, when the onion is translucent and beginning to brown on the edges, add the cabbage and season generously with salt and pepper. About 5 minutes later, when the cabbage begins to soften and become lighter in color, add the Bone Broth, vinegar, and rosemary. Cover the pan and allow the vegetables to steam for 3 to 5 minutes, then reduce the heat to low and cook, uncovered, until the cabbage is softened and almost no liquid remains, approximately 10 to 15 minutes.

olive oil & garlic spaghetti

PREP TIME **5 MINS** • COOK TIME **45 TO 50 MINS** • SERVINGS **4**

1 large spaghetti squash

1 tablespoon cooking fat*

sea salt and black pepper to taste

2 teaspoons granulated garlic

1 teaspoon dried oregano

1/2 cup kalamata or oil-cured black olives (pictured), halved

1/4 cup extra-virgin olive oil, to finish

Preheat the oven to 375°F.

Slice the spaghetti squash in half lengthwise. Scoop the seeds and inner membranes out of the hollows, then place both halves face down on a rimmed baking sheet. Roast for 35 to 45 minutes or until the flesh of the squash becomes translucent and the skin begins to soften and separate from the noodles that make up the inside. Allow the squash to cool enough that you can handle it, then scoop out the flesh into a large, high-sided skillet or sauté pan. Add the cooking fat to keep it from sticking, and toss the squash to coat it evenly with the fat in the pan.

Set the skillet over medium heat, then season the squash with the salt and pepper, garlic, and oregano. Add the olives and toss to combine. Allow the squash to heat through, then remove it from the heat and finish it with the olive oil, tossing again to combine it.

Serve warm as a side dish or add sliced chicken, baked fish, or mini meatballs to make it a complete meal.

INGREDIENT TIP
*Refer to page 228 to see which fats are best for cooking.

CHEF NOTE
This recipe is quick and easy if you roast the spaghetti squash ahead of time and have it ready to go into the skillet with the rest of the ingredients when it's time to eat. That will cut your cooking time down to 10 minutes! ●

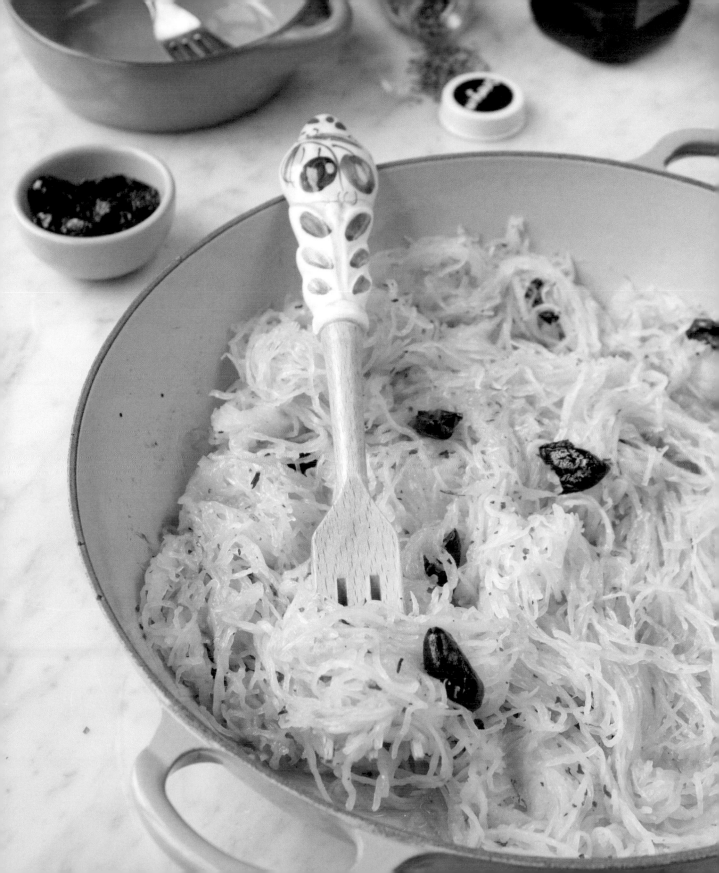

roasted butternut squash mash

PREP TIME **15 MINS** • COOK TIME **30 TO 35 MINS** • SERVINGS **4**

NUTS

EGGS

NIGHTSHADES

FODMAPS

SEAFOOD

1 large butternut squash

5 tablespoons ghee or coconut oil, divided

sea salt

1/4 cup full-fat coconut milk, canned* or homemade (page 210)

2 to 4 tablespoons warm water

a few fresh sage leaves

Preheat the oven to 350°F.

Peel the squash, cut it in half, and remove the seeds. Chop into 1-inch pieces and place on 2 rimmed baking sheets. Pour 1 tablespoon of the ghee or coconut oil over each baking sheet and toss the squash pieces with the oil to coat them well. Season liberally with salt. Roast for 30 to 35 minutes or until the squash is soft but not overly browned.

Place the squash in a food processor and add 2 tablespoons of the ghee or coconut oil, the coconut milk, and warm water 1 tablespoon at a time until the puree reaches a smooth consistency, stopping to scrape the sides of the bowl as necessary. This will take a few minutes. Add salt to taste.

In a small skillet, heat the remaining 1 tablespoon of the ghee or coconut oil. When the ghee is hot, add the sage leaves to the pan and fry for 1 minute per side or until the sage becomes dark green and crispy.

This side is a perfect complement to the Cinnamon & Fennel Braised Pork on page 84.

INGREDIENT TIP
*Check out pages 226–227 for a list of recommended brands.

FODMAP-FREE?
Omit the coconut milk and add more warm water as needed.

CHANGE IT UP
Use steamed or roasted carrots instead of squash. ●

Use 4 medium sweet potatoes, peeled and cut into 1/2-inch pieces, instead of butternut squash.

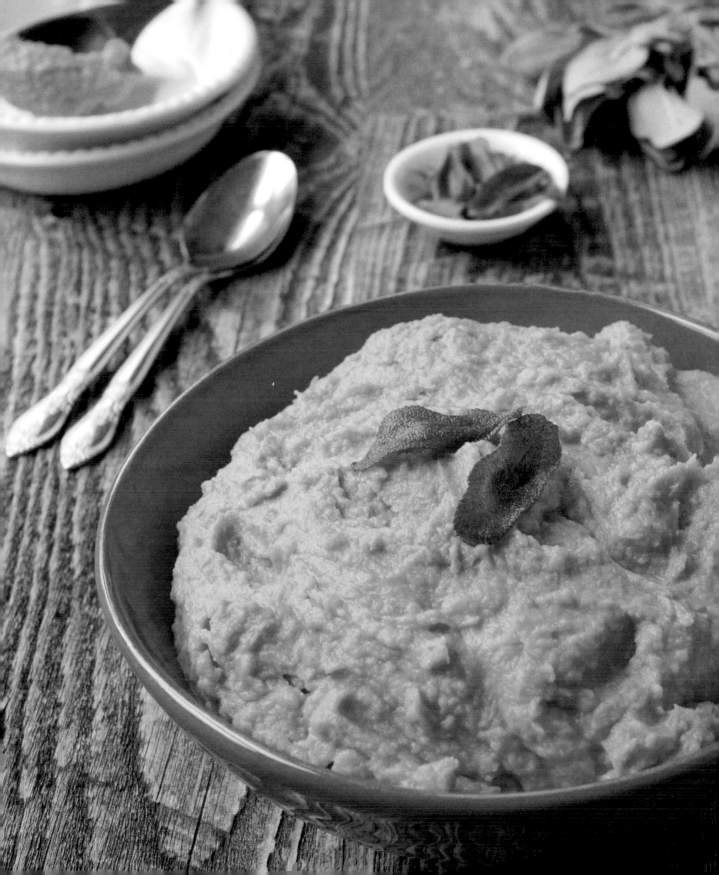

broccoli double take

PREP TIME **5 MINS** • COOK TIME **20 MINS** • SERVINGS **4**

NUTS

EGGS

NIGHTSHADES

FODMAPS

SEAFOOD

1 large head broccoli (with long stem intact)

4 tablespoons ghee or coconut oil, divided

sea salt and black pepper

1/2 teaspoon onion powder

1/2 teaspoon granulated garlic

Preheat the oven to 350°F. Set up a pot with 1 to 2 inches of water and a steamer basket.

Slice the long, thick stem off of the broccoli and cut it into 2-inch lengths.

Remove the largest florets and stalks from the head of the broccoli and slice them in half lengthwise. Continue until only small stalks remain at the top of the head. These remaining pieces should be small enough that slicing them in half lengthwise would be quite tricky. Remove these stalks and do not slice them in half.

Brush a rimmed baking sheet with 1 tablespoon of the ghee and place the long, halved stalks of broccoli on the baking sheet. Season generously with salt and pepper and bake for 10 minutes. Flip them over and bake until they begin to brown, about 10 minutes more.

While the long stalks bake, place the stems and smaller stalks in the steamer pot and steam for 10 minutes or until fork-tender. Once the stalks are cooked through, place them in a food processor and blend with the remaining 3 tablespoons of ghee, onion powder, and granulated garlic, and add salt and pepper to taste.

Serve the roasted stalks on top of the puree.

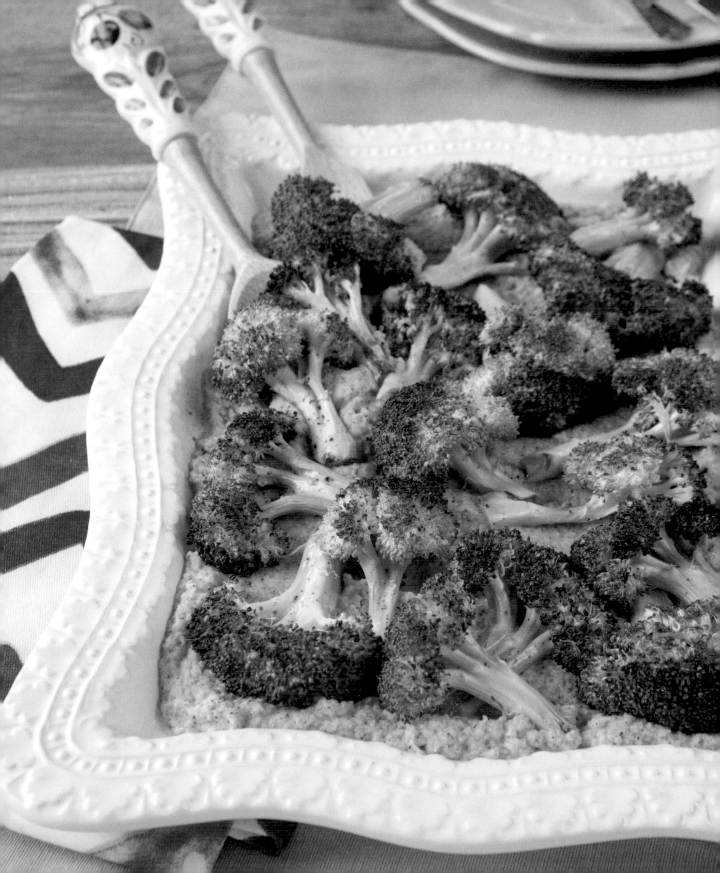

roasted garlic parsnip mash

PREP TIME **15 MINS** • COOK TIME **45 MINS** • SERVINGS **4**

NUTS

EGGS

NIGHTSHADES

FODMAPS

SEAFOOD

1 head garlic

1/4 cup plus 2 tablespoons ghee or coconut oil, divided

6 large parsnips, peeled and cut into 1-inch pieces

1 teaspoon sea salt

1/2 teaspoon black pepper

2 tablespoons sliced green onion (scallion), for garnish (optional)

Roast the garlic: Preheat the oven to 350°F. Slice the top and bottom off of the garlic bulb, then top with 2 tablespoons of the ghee. Wrap securely in aluminum foil and bake for approximately 40 minutes. Remove from the oven and, when cool enough to handle, gently squeeze the roasted cloves from the bulb. They should slide out easily.

While the garlic roasts, place the parsnips in a pot and cover with water by 1 inch. Bring to a boil and cook for 10 to 15 minutes or until the parsnips are fork-tender. Drain the water from the pan and let the parsnips sit for 5 minutes to let the extra moisture evaporate.

Place the parsnips, the remaining 1/4 cup of ghee, 8 cloves of the roasted garlic, salt, and pepper in a food processor and process until creamy, about 5 minutes, scraping down the sides often.

Garnish with sliced green onion if desired.

CHEF NOTE
Fold 1 to 2 tablespoons of freshly chopped herbs into the mash for a change of pace—basil pairs well with Italian-style dishes, and cilantro or parsley works well with other cuisines.

KITCHEN TIP
Preparing roasted garlic ahead of time makes this recipe a much quicker side dish for a weeknight meal! ●

Use 4 medium sweet potatoes, peeled and cut into 1/2-inch pieces, instead of parsnips.

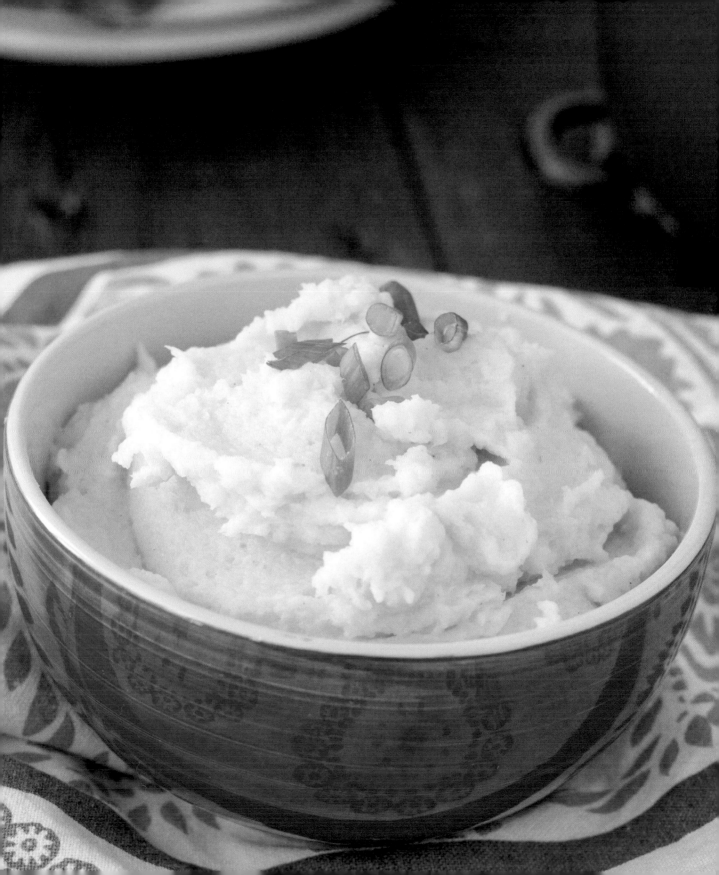

caramelized brussels sprouts & onions

PREP TIME **10 MINS** • COOK TIME **20 TO 25 MINS** • SERVINGS **4**

NUTS

EGGS

NIGHTSHADES

FODMAPS

SEAFOOD

6 to 8 slices bacon, chopped
1/2 red onion, diced (1 cup)
1 pound Brussels sprouts
sea salt and black pepper

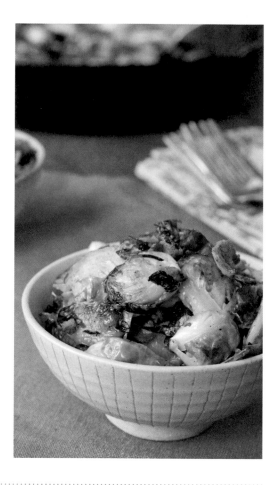

Over medium-high heat, cook the bacon in a skillet until cooked through but not crispy, about 4 to 5 minutes. Add the red onion and cook for 2 to 3 minutes or until soft. While the bacon and onion cook, cut off the bottom of each Brussels sprout and then slice each sprout into 4 pieces. Add the Brussels sprouts to the pan with the bacon and toss to thoroughly coat with the bacon fat.

Season lightly with salt and pepper. Let the sprouts cook without stirring for 3 to 5 minutes or until they start to develop a deep brown, caramelized color. Stir the sprouts and then cook for another 2 to 3 minutes, undisturbed, before stirring again. Continue to cook this way for a total of 8 to 10 minutes or until the sprouts are soft. Check for seasoning and add more salt or pepper if needed.

spiced applesauce

PREP TIME **10 MINS** • COOK TIME **30 MINS** • SERVINGS **4**

4 green apples, peeled and
    diced
1/4 cup water
2 pinches ground nutmeg
2 pinches ground allspice
1 pinch ground cloves
1/2 teaspoon ground
    cinnamon
1 cinnamon stick

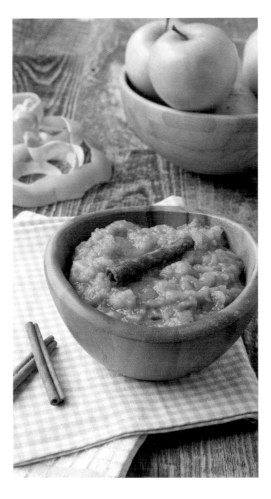

NUTS

EGGS

NIGHTSHADES

FODMAPS

SEAFOOD

CHEF NOTE
Blending/puréeing
is not required for
a soft applesauce;
simply continue
to cook the
apples until they
completely soften.

CHANGE IT UP
Add some curls of
orange zest for a
twist on the flavor
of this sauce. ●

Place all the ingredients in a
saucepan. Bring to a simmer over
medium-low heat and simmer for
30 minutes or until the apples are
cooked and become soft to your
desired texture, chunky or smooth.
Remove the cinnamon stick before
serving or storing.

creamy cucumber salad

PREP TIME **10 MINS** • SERVINGS **4**

NUTS

EGGS

NIGHTSHADES

FODMAPS

SEAFOOD

2 large cucumbers, peeled and sliced into 1/8-inch rounds

sea salt and black pepper

juice of 1 lemon

3 tablespoons chopped fresh dill, plus a sprig for optional garnish

1/3 cup full-fat coconut milk, canned* or homemade (page 210)

1 small clove garlic, minced or grated

Place the cucumber slices in a mixing bowl and season lightly with salt and pepper. In a small mixing bowl, whisk together the lemon juice, dill, coconut milk, and garlic. Season with salt and pepper to taste. Pour the creamy dressing over the cucumber slices and toss to combine. Garnish with a sprig of dill if desired.

This salad can be eaten immediately or after chilling for several hours or overnight in the refrigerator.

INGREDIENT TIP
*Check out pages 226–227 for a list of recommended brands. ●

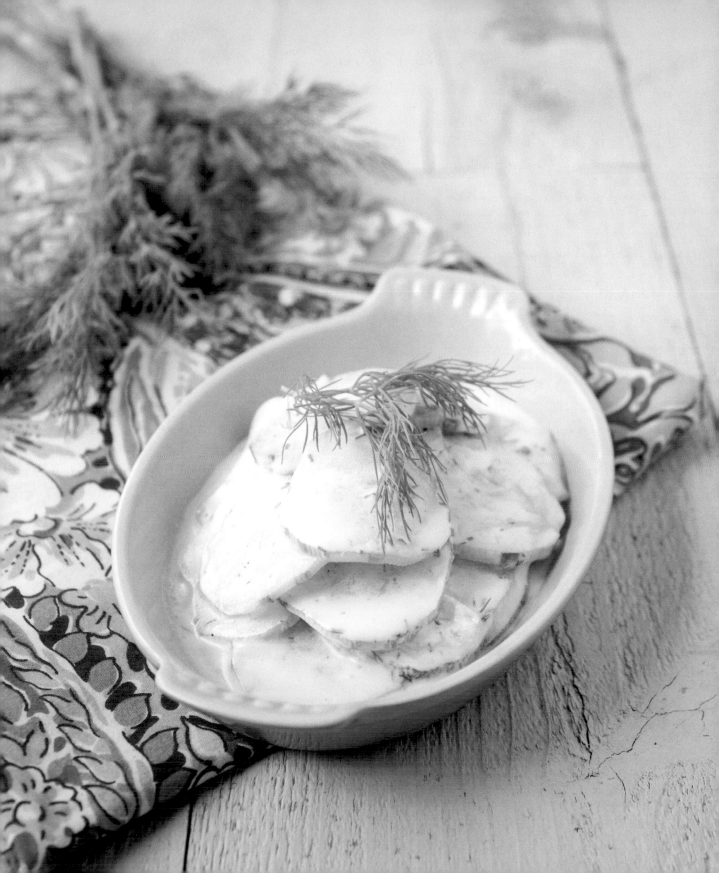

green bean casserole

PREP TIME **5 MINS (+ 30 MINS TO MAKE THE SOUP)** • COOK TIME **35 MINS** • SERVINGS **4 TO 6**

NUTS

EGGS

NIGHTSHADES

FODMAPS

SEAFOOD

1 teaspoon bacon fat
or ghee

1 large shallot, thinly sliced
(1/4 cup)

1 1/2 to 2 pounds green
beans, trimmed

1 1/2 cups Creamy
Mushroom Soup
(page 132)

1/2 cup almond meal* or
other nut meal

sea salt and black pepper

Preheat the oven to 350°F.

In a small skillet over medium heat, melt the
bacon fat, then cook the shallots in the fat until
translucent and slightly browned on the edges,
about 5 minutes.

Roughly chop the green beans and place them
in a 9-by-13-inch baking dish. Pour the Creamy
Mushroom Soup over the green beans, then
top evenly with the almond meal. Sprinkle
the top with salt and pepper and then evenly
distribute the shallots across the top. Bake
for 20 to 30 minutes or until the sides of the
casserole are bubbling.

INGREDIENT TIP
*Check out pages 226–227 for a list of
recommended brands. ●

Make the Creamy Mushroom Soup called for in this
recipe with Vegetable Broth (page 208) instead of
Beef Broth.

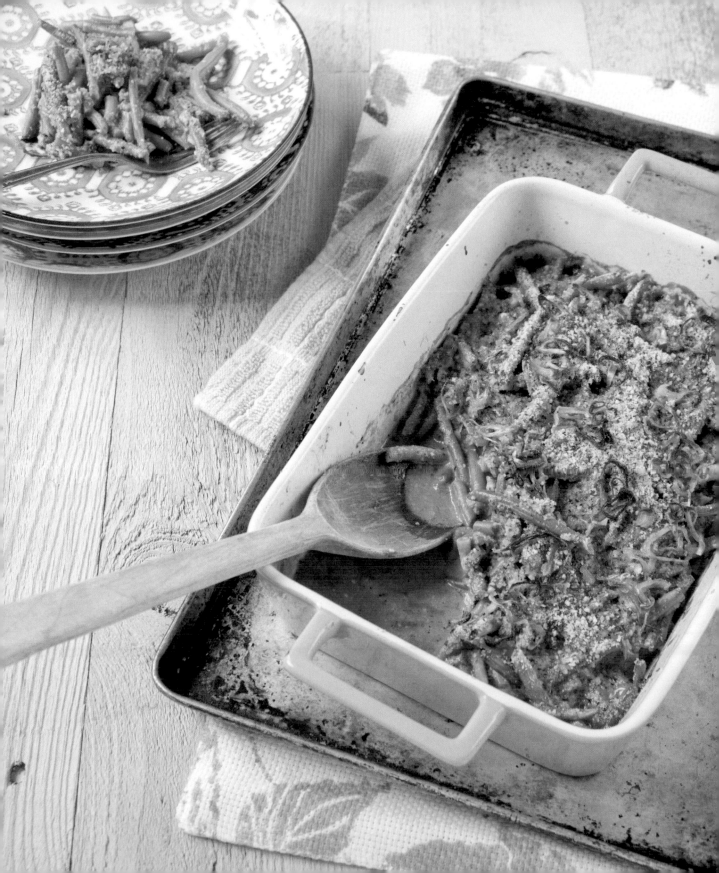

mini sweet potato flatbreads

PREP TIME **15 MINS**   •   COOK TIME **15 MINS**   •   SERVINGS **4**   •   YIELD **16 (4-INCH) ROUNDS**

NUTS

EGGS

NIGHTSHADES

FODMAPS

SEAFOOD

6 teaspoons gelatin*

5 tablespoons coconut flour**

2 cups steamed and mashed sweet potato (both orange and white sweet potatoes were used in the breads pictured)

4 eggs

1/4 cup ghee, butter, or coconut oil

1 teaspoon sea salt

Preheat the oven to 400°F. Line two baking sheets with parchment paper.

Combine all the ingredients in a bowl or food processor and mix until the ingredients are thoroughly combined and a sticky dough forms. Wet your hands and separate the dough into 16 equal portions. Form each portion into a ball and place on the prepared baking sheets. Press out each round to a 4-inch diameter circle, wetting your hands when the mixture begins to stick.

Bake until slightly browned on the edges, about 15 minutes, flipping the flatbreads halfway through.

INGREDIENT TIP
*I recommend Great Lakes brand grass-fed gelatin with the orange/red label. Note that the green label variety can be used in smoothies but it doesn't work for this recipe because it will not gel.

**See pages 226-227 for recommended brands.

CHEF NOTE
If your steamed sweet potatoes seem to contain more water, yielding a loose dough, add more coconut flour to the batter, 1 teaspoon at a time, until the batter firms up. ●

 This recipe is only suitable if you are following Energy Modifications.

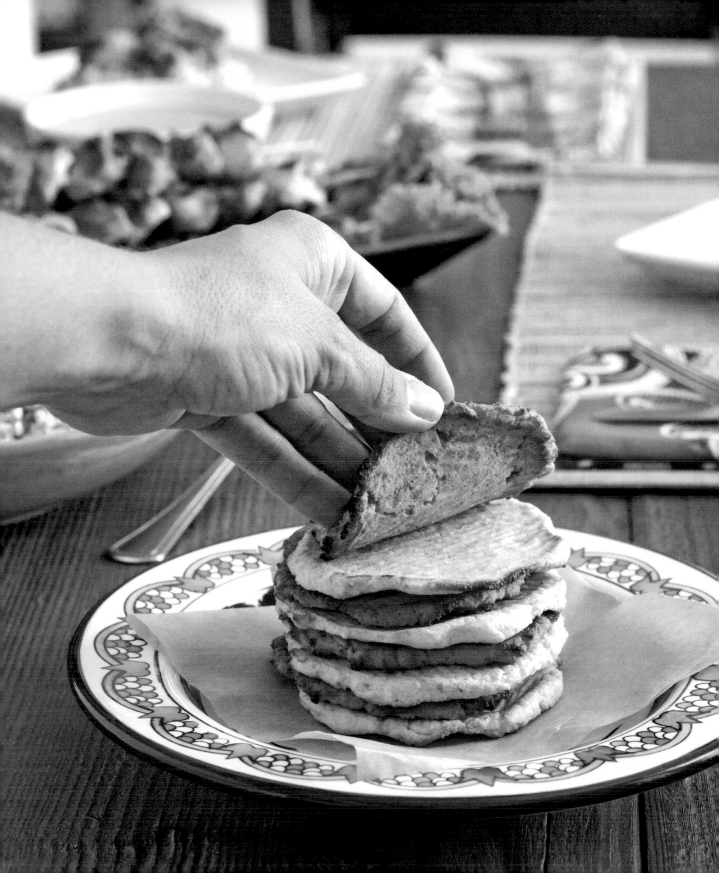

fennel & bacon sweet potato salad

PREP TIME **20 MINS** • COOK TIME **20 MINS** • SERVINGS **4 TO 6**

NUTS
EGGS
NIGHTSHADES
FODMAPS
SEAFOOD

4 medium sweet potatoes, peeled and cut into 1-inch cubes (4 cups)

6 slices bacon

1/2 medium red onion, diced (1/2 cup)

2 green onions (scallions), sliced (1/4 cup)

1/2 cup thinly sliced fennel bulb

3/4 cup Healthy Homemade Mayonnaise (page 219)

1 tablespoon apple cider vinegar*

1 teaspoon sea salt

1/4 teaspoon black pepper

Place the sweet potatoes in a large pot and add water to cover them by about 1 inch. Bring to a boil and cook for about 10 minutes or until fork-tender. Drain the potatoes and set aside to cool slightly.

Cook the bacon in a skillet over medium heat until the fat has rendered off, about 8 to 10 minutes. Remove the bacon from the pan and drain on paper towels. When the bacon is cool, chop it. (Reserve the bacon fat for another use.)

In a large bowl, combine the red and green onions, fennel, and bacon. In a small bowl, mix together the Mayonnaise, vinegar, salt, and pepper. Add the potatoes to the bowl with the onions and fennel and toss lightly to mix. Gently fold in the mayonnaise mixture until well combined. Check for seasoning and, if needed, add more salt and pepper to taste. Serve warm or chill for deeper flavor.

This salad pairs perfectly with the Coffee & Cocoa Rubbed Ribs, page 100.

INGREDIENT TIP
*Check out pages 226–227 for a list of recommended brands. ●

 This recipe is only suitable if you are following Energy Modifications.

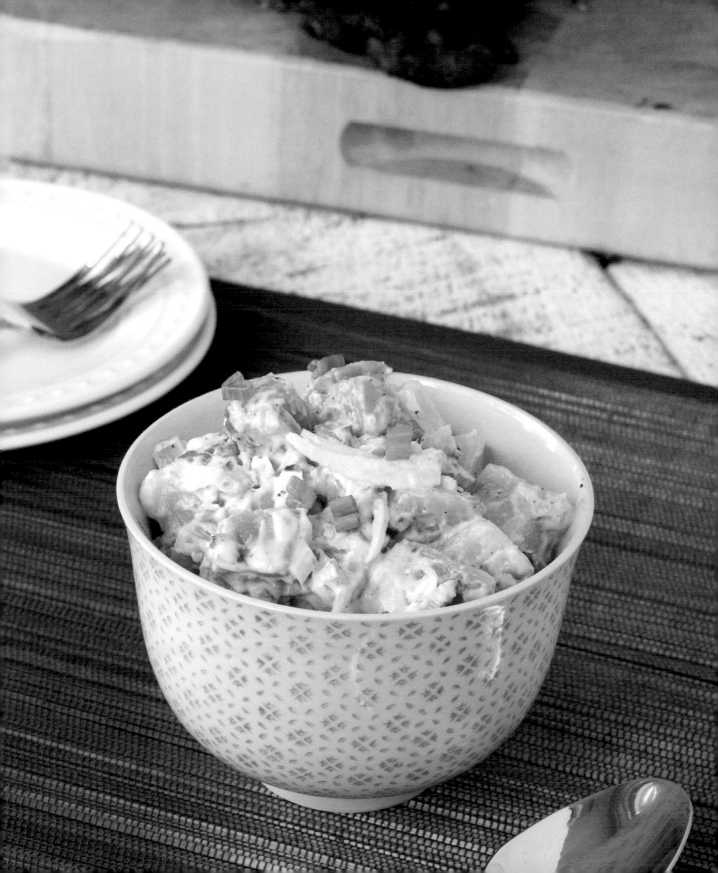

seasoned sweet potato fries

PREP TIME **10 MINS** • COOK TIME **30 MINS** • SERVINGS **2**

NUTS

EGGS

NIGHTSHADES

FODMAPS

SEAFOOD

2 medium sweet potatoes, peeled (do not rinse)

1 tablespoon coconut oil or other cooking fat,* melted

1 teaspoon ground cumin

1 teaspoon granulated garlic

1/2 teaspoon ground cinnamon

1/2 teaspoon black pepper

1/4 teaspoon sea salt, or more to taste

Sweetener-Free Ketchup (page 216), for serving (optional)

Position 2 oven racks in the top third of the oven and preheat the oven to 450°F. Line 2 rimmed baking sheets with parchment paper.

Cut the sweet potatoes into 1/4-inch-thick sticks.

In a medium bowl, combine the melted coconut oil and the spices. Toss the sweet potatoes in the coconut oil mixture until evenly coated. Place the sweet potatoes on the prepared baking sheets in a single layer, spaced evenly apart. Bake in the upper part of the oven for 15 minutes. Flip over the sweet potatoes and switch the position of the baking sheets if one is browning faster than the other. Cook for an additional 10 to 15 minutes or until the edges of the fries are dark golden brown. Season with additional salt, if needed, while the fries are still warm, and serve with Ketchup, if desired.

INGREDIENT TIP
*See page 228 for a list of recommended cooking fats.

NIGHTSHADE FREE?
Dip in Creamy Ranch Dressing (page 204) instead of ketchup! ●

This recipe is only suitable if you are following Energy Modifications.

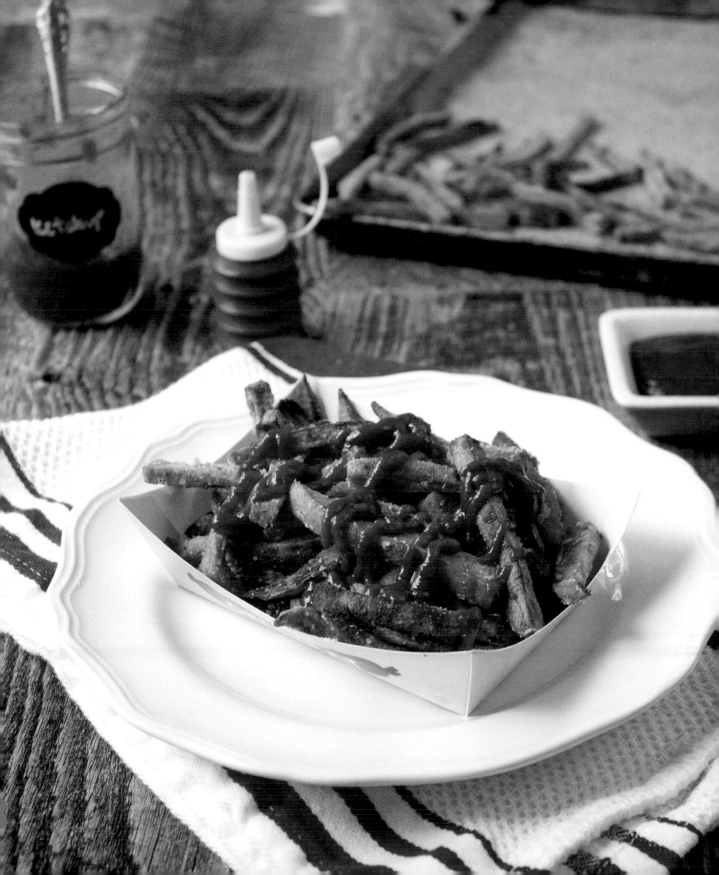

NUTS

EGGS

NIGHTSHADES

FODMAPS

SEAFOOD

pesto deviled eggs

PREP TIME **10 MINS** • SERVINGS **4**

8 hard-boiled eggs, peeled

1/3 cup Healthy Homemade
   Mayonnaise (page 219)

1 teaspoon gluten-free
   Dijon mustard*

1/8 teaspoon paprika

1/4 cup Spinach & Walnut
   Pesto (page 207)

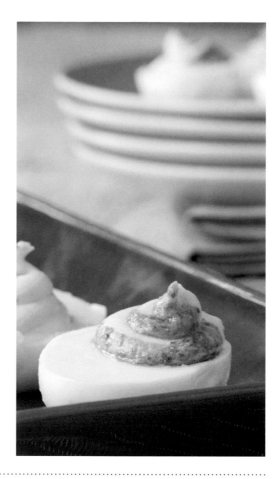

INGREDIENT TIP
*Check out pages
226–227 for a list
of recommended
brands. ●

Cut each hard-boiled egg in half lengthwise and remove the yolks. Place the yolks in a food processor or bowl with the Mayonnaise, mustard, and paprika and mix until creamy and completely combined.

Fill one side of a pastry bag or plastic sandwich bag with the yolk-mayonnaise mixture and the other side with the pesto—this will create a swirl effect when piped into the egg whites. If using a sandwich bag, snip about 1/2 inch off the corner of the bag. Using a circular motion, fill the egg whites.

Keep chilled until ready to serve.

dill crackers

PREP TIME **10 MIN (+ 20 MINS TO CHILL)** • COOK TIME **10 TO 12 MINS**
• YIELD **3 TO 4 DOZEN CRACKERS**

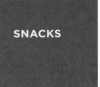

3 eggs

3 tablespoons ghee or coconut oil

6 tablespoons cold water

1 teaspoon onion powder

1 teaspoon granulated garlic

1 teaspoon chopped fresh dill

1/2 teaspoon sea salt

1/2 teaspoon black pepper

2 tablespoons arrowroot flour

1 cup coconut flour*

NUTS

EGGS

NIGHTSHADES

FODMAPS

SEAFOOD

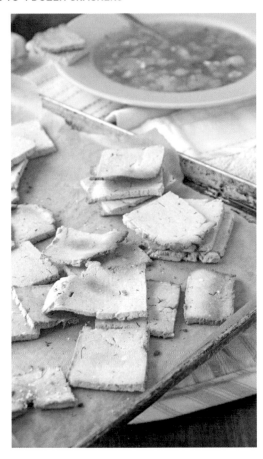

INGREDIENT TIP
*Check out pages 226–227 for a list of recommended brands. ●

Whisk together the eggs, ghee, water, onion powder, granulated garlic, dill, salt, and pepper. Sift the arrowroot flour and coconut flour into the wet mixture and combine—first with a large spoon, then with your hands—until well incorporated. Form the mixture into 2 balls and wrap each ball tightly with plastic wrap. Chill the dough for at least 20 minutes.

Preheat the oven to 350°F.

After the dough has chilled, roll one ball between 2 sheets of parchment paper with a rolling pin until it's an even 1/8-inch-thick rectangle. Repeat with the second ball of dough. Transfer the sheets of dough on the parchment to 2 separate sheet pans and slice into crackers of your desired size and shape.

Bake for 10 to 12 minutes or until the edges of the crackers are golden brown. If you don't have 2 sheet pans, you can bake the crackers in 2 batches.

sunbutter

PREP TIME **25 MINS** • COOK TIME **5 MINS** • YIELD **2 CUPS**

NUTS

EGGS

NIGHTSHADES

FODMAPS

SEAFOOD

3 cups raw, unsalted sunflower seeds

1/2 to 1 teaspoon sea salt, or to taste

3 tablespoons coconut butter,* melted

1 tablespoon coconut oil, melted

1 tablespoon pure vanilla extract (optional)

Toast the sunflower seeds in a large skillet over low heat, stirring frequently. Remove from the heat when about half of the seeds are slightly browned. Be careful not to overtoast the seeds, as this will remove too much moisture and the sunbutter won't get creamy. Remove the seeds from the pan and let cool for about 5 minutes.

Pour the toasted sunflower seeds and 1/2 teaspoon of salt into a food processor and begin to process, stopping to scrape down the sides often. The seeds will first produce a fine meal, and after about 10 minutes the mixture will start to clump together. About 15 minutes in, the consistency will be that of very thick peanut butter. Add the coconut butter, coconut oil, and vanilla and process for another 5 to 7 minutes or until creamy. Taste and add more salt if desired. The mixture will firm up as it cools and will be thick if kept in the refrigerator.

INGREDIENT TIP
*Check out pages 226–227 for a list of recommended brands. ●

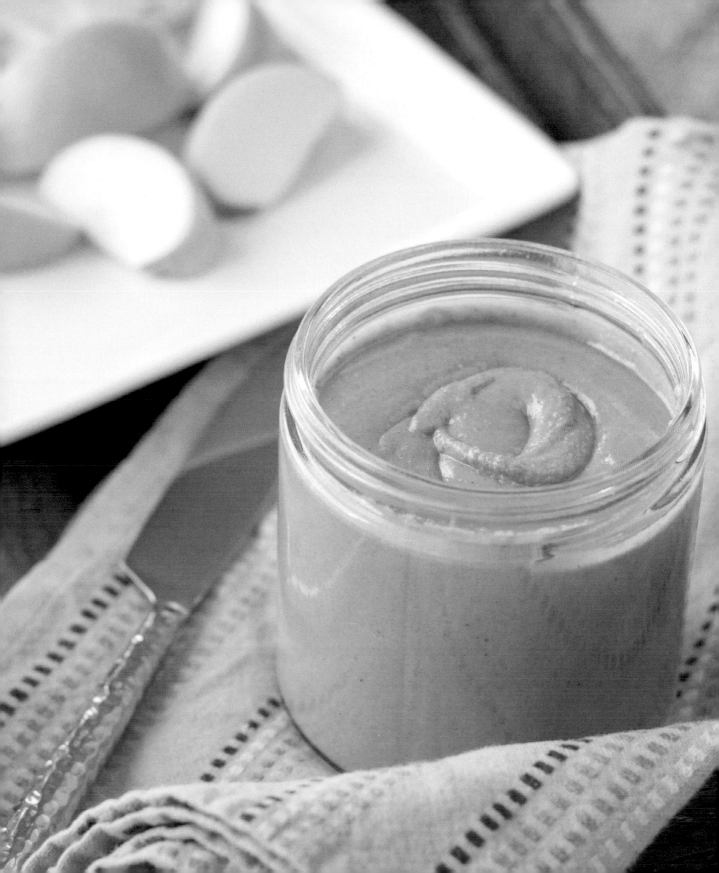

"buttermilk" buns

PREP TIME **10 MINS** • COOK TIME **10 TO 15 MINS** • SERVINGS **4** • YIELD **8 BUNS**

NUTS
EGGS
NIGHTSHADES
FODMAPS
SEAFOOD

1/4 cup full-fat coconut milk, canned* or homemade (page 210)

1 tablespoon apple cider vinegar*

2 teaspoons gelatin

4 eggs, cold

1/4 cup coconut flour,* sifted

1/4 cup almond flour*

1 teaspoon baking soda

1/2 teaspoon sea salt

Preheat the oven to 350°F. Line a baking sheet with parchment paper.

Whisk together the coconut milk, apple cider vinegar, and gelatin in a small bowl and let sit for 5 minutes.

In a medium bowl, whisk together the eggs, coconut milk mixture, coconut flour, almond flour, baking soda, and salt. Let sit for 5 minutes. The consistency of the batter should be similar to that of a thick pancake batter—it should not spread much on its own when put on the baking sheet. If the batter seems too runny, add 1 tablespoon of sifted coconut flour and blend well.

Scoop 3 tablespoons of the batter onto the prepared baking sheet and gently spread it into 3-inch circles. Bake for 10 to 15 minutes or until the buns feel springy in the center when gently pressed.

These buns may be reheated the next day in a toaster or toaster oven.

INGREDIENT TIP
*Check out pages 226–227 for a list of recommended brands. ●

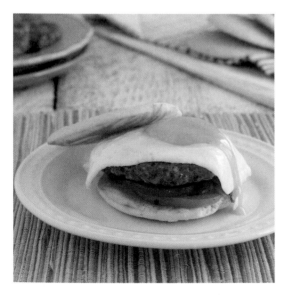

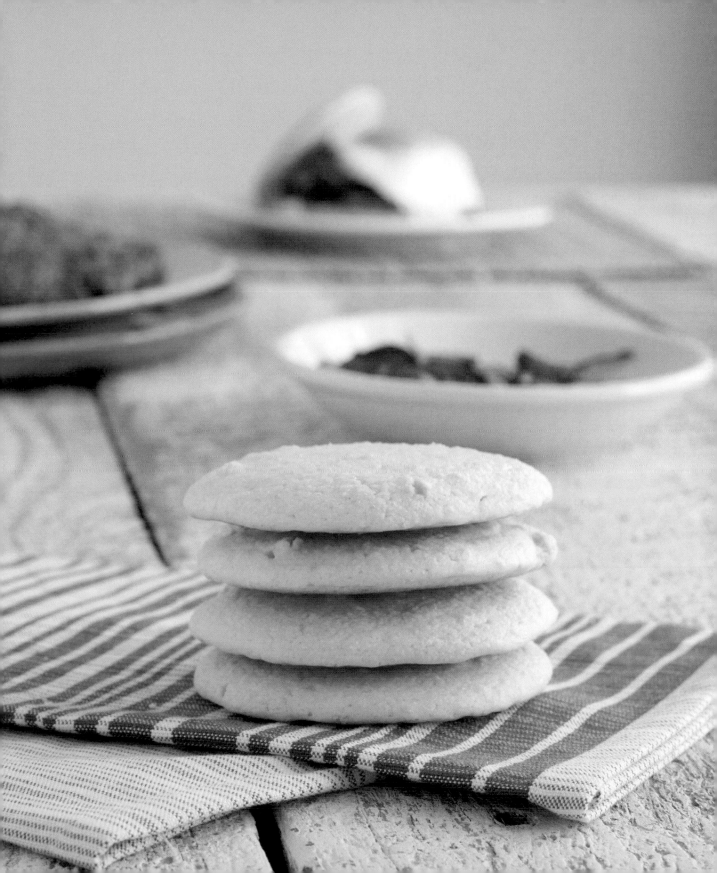

celery root cakes

PREP TIME **10 MINS** • COOK TIME **10 MINS** • SERVINGS **6** • YIELD **12 SMALL CAKES**

NUTS
EGGS
NIGHTSHADES
FODMAPS
SEAFOOD

1 egg
1/2 teaspoon sea salt
1/2 teaspoon black pepper
1/2 teaspoon granulated garlic
1 large celery root, peeled and shredded (2 cups)
coconut oil or other cooking fat* for pan frying

INGREDIENT TIP
*Refer to page 228 to see which fats are best for cooking. ●

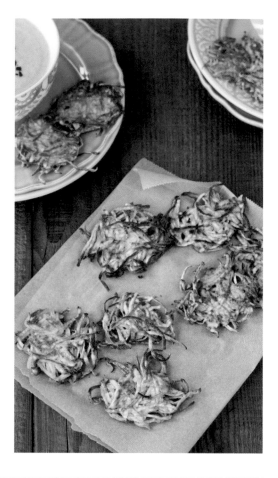

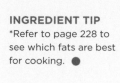

In a large mixing bowl, whisk the egg with the seasonings, then add the celery root and mix together until the celery root is well coated.

In a large skillet over medium-high heat, melt enough cooking fat to cover the entire bottom of your skillet in a very thin layer. When the skillet is hot, form the cakes. (You want the oil to be hot enough to brown the celery root quickly, but not hot enough to burn it before it cooks together enough for you to flip the cake over.) I recommend cooking a small test cake before you make the whole batch.

Form about 2 tablespoons of the mixture into a loose ball and press into a thin, even layer in the bottom of the skillet. Repeat with the rest of the mixture. Fry until browned on one side, about 1 minute, and then quickly flip over to cook for another 1 minute on the other side. Remove and place on a towel-lined plate. These are best if eaten immediately.

Use shredded sweet potato instead of celery root and fry over medium heat for 3 minutes per side.

sundried tomato hummus

PREP TIME **10 MINS** • SERVINGS **8** • YIELD **2 CUPS**

4 cups cauliflower florets, steamed

2 tablespoons sesame tahini, plus more if desired

1/4 cup + 1 tablespoon extra-virgin olive oil, plus more if desired

1 small clove garlic, minced

zest and juice of 1 lemon

pinch of ground cumin

sea salt and black pepper to taste

6 sundried tomatoes, diced, plus more for garnish

paprika, for garnish

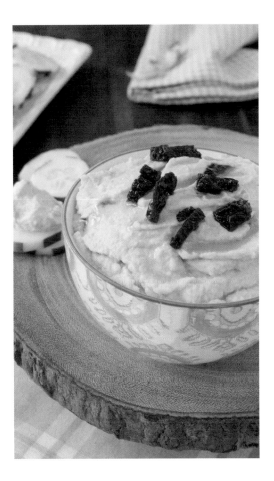

NUTS

EGGS

NIGHTSHADES

FODMAPS

SEAFOOD

In a food processor, combine the cauliflower, tahini, 1/4 cup of the olive oil, garlic, lemon juice, and cumin until smooth. Season with salt and pepper and add more tahini or olive oil to taste. Add the sundried tomatoes and pulse to combine.

Scoop out the hummus from the food processor and garnish with lemon zest, the additional 1 tablespoon of olive oil, a sprinkling of paprika, and additional diced sundried tomatoes.

Serve with your choice of sliced fresh vegetables and olives.

herb almond "cheese" spread

PREP TIME **8 HRS + 10 MINS** • YIELD **2 CUPS**

NUTS
EGGS
NIGHTSHADES
FODMAPS
SEAFOOD

1 cup raw almonds

2 1/4 cups water, divided

5 tablespoons extra-virgin olive oil

1/4 cup fresh lemon juice (2 lemons)

1 clove garlic, minced or grated

2 tablespoons minced fresh chives

sea salt and black pepper to taste

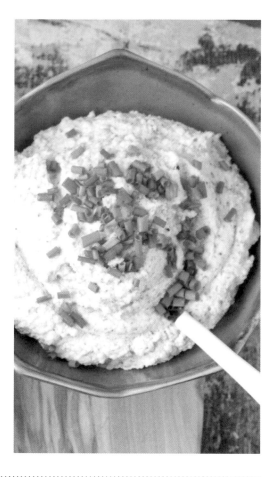

Place the almonds and 2 cups of the water in a glass or other nonporous container and let them soak, covered, in a dark place, overnight or for 8 hours.

Drain and rinse the almonds, then place them in a food processor along with the remaining 1/4 cup water and the rest of the ingredients. Process until smooth and creamy, stopping occasionally to scrape down the sides, about 5 minutes total.

If you'd like a lighter texture, add warm water, 1 tablespoon at a time, until you achieve the desired consistency.

smoky lime nut mix

PREP TIME **10 MINS** • COOK TIME **25 MINS** • SERVINGS **6** • YIELD **1 1/2 CUPS**

SNACKS

1/2 cup raw almonds

1/2 cup raw walnuts

1/2 cup raw pecans

juice of 1/2 lime

1 1/2 tablespoons coconut oil, melted

2 teaspoons Smoky Spice Blend (page 222)

zest of 1 lime

sea salt to taste

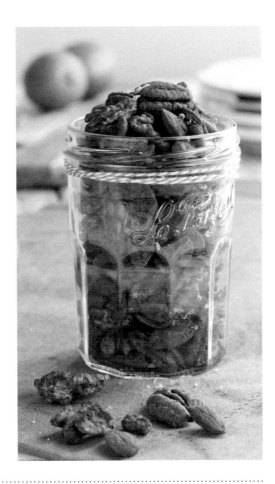

NUTS

EGGS

NIGHTSHADES

FODMAPS

SEAFOOD

Preheat the oven to 275°F.

In a medium bowl, combine the nuts and lime juice and toss to coat. Let sit for at least 5 minutes.

In a small bowl, combine the melted coconut oil, Spice Blend, and lime zest.

Toss the nuts in the lime juice one more time to coat, then drain the excess lime juice from the bowl. Add the coconut oil mixture and toss to completely coat the mixed nuts. Season with salt to taste. Spread the nuts out in a single layer on a rimmed baking sheet and bake for 20 to 25 minutes or until toasted. Place in a glass jar and store in the refrigerator for up to 3 weeks. Note: A white film may appear on the nut mix when it is refrigerated, as coconut oil becomes solid when cold. This film will disappear when the nut mix reaches room temperature.

salt & vinegar kale chips

PREP TIME **10 MINS** • COOK TIME **20 MINS, + 20 MINS EXTRA DRYING TIME IF NEEDED** • SERVINGS **4 TO 6**

NUTS

EGGS

NIGHTSHADES

FODMAPS

SEAFOOD

3 tablespoons coconut oil, melted

1/2 cup almond or other nut or seed meal*

1/2 cup nutritional yeast*

1/4 cup apple cider vinegar*

1 teaspoon sea salt

1 large bunch kale

Preheat the oven to 350°F.

In a large mixing bowl, combine the coconut oil, almond meal, nutritional yeast, vinegar, and salt. Rinse the kale and dry it very well by patting it with paper towels or clean kitchen towels, then hold the end of each stem and pull the leaves off of the stem. Tear very large leaves into smaller pieces, then place the kale in the bowl with the topping mixture. Massage the mixture into the kale leaves, then spread the kale in a single layer on a baking sheet. You will likely need to use 2 pans or bake the kale chips in 2 batches.

Bake for 15 to 20 minutes or until the kale becomes crispy but not browned. If after 20 minutes of baking the kale still seems a bit soggy (which often happens if the kale was not completely dry before baking), simply turn off the oven and leave the kale in the oven while it cools for an additional 20 minutes. This will give the kale more time to dry out.

INGREDIENT TIP
*Check out pages 226–227 for a list of recommended brands.

NUT-FREE?
Omit the nut meal. ●

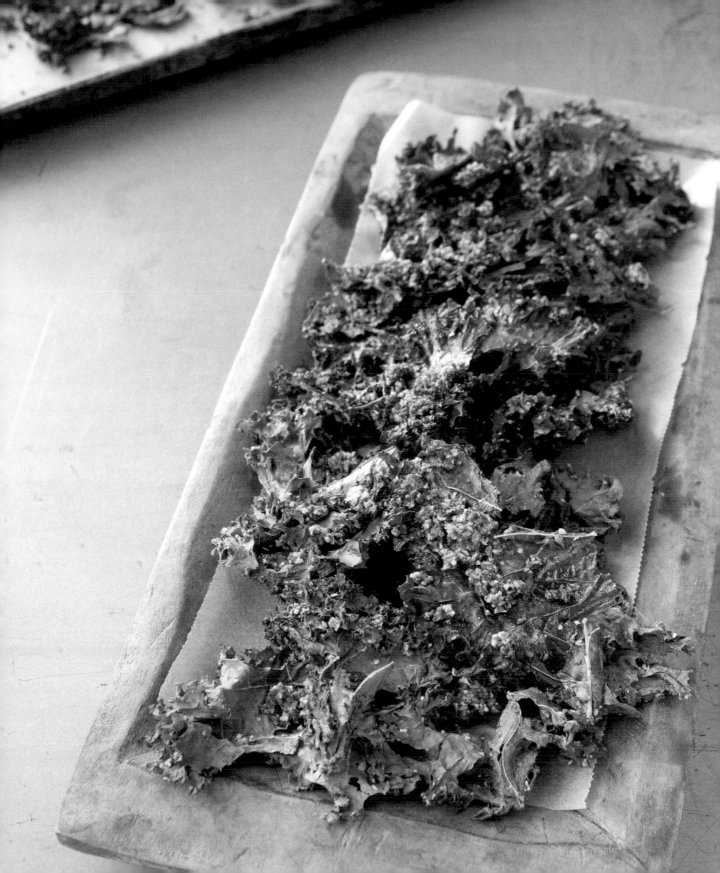

turkey jerky

PREP TIME **10 MINS + OVERNIGHT MARINATING** • COOK TIME **3 TO 4 HRS** • SERVINGS **8**

2 pounds boneless, skinless turkey breast (frozen for 1 to 2 hours)

Choose one marinade below, or use 4 pounds total and make both flavor options.

CHINESE FIVE SPICE JERKY OPTION

1/2 cup coconut aminos*

1 tablespoon fish sauce*

1/2 teaspoon Chinese Five-Spice powder

1 teaspoon sea salt

CHILI-GARLIC JERKY OPTION

1/2 cup clean ingredient hot sauce*

juice of 1 lime

1 teaspoon granulated garlic

1/2 teaspoon sea salt

In a medium bowl, whisk together the ingredients for the marinade flavoring of your choice. Taste and adjust the seasonings as desired; it should taste stronger than you want the finished jerky to taste.

Remove the turkey breast from the freezer—you want it to be firm enough to cut into thin slices, but not completely frozen. Cutting against the grain, very thinly slice the turkey breast into 1/8-inch slices using a sharp knife, electric carving knife, or meat slicer.

Place the sliced meat in the marinade and refrigerate overnight.

Preheat the oven to 200°F. Place oven-safe baking racks on top of 2 foil-lined rimmed baking sheets.

Remove the meat from the refrigerator and place the racks at least 1/2-inch apart. Bake for 3 to 4 hours or until the jerky reaches the desired level of dryness, keeping in mind that it will harden a bit as it cools.

If you have a dehydrator, you can dehydrate the marinated turkey strips on low for 3 to 4 hours or until dry to your texture preference. Store refrigerated in an airtight glass container or bag for up to 2 weeks.

INGREDIENT TIP
*Check out pages 226–227 for a list of recommended brands. ●

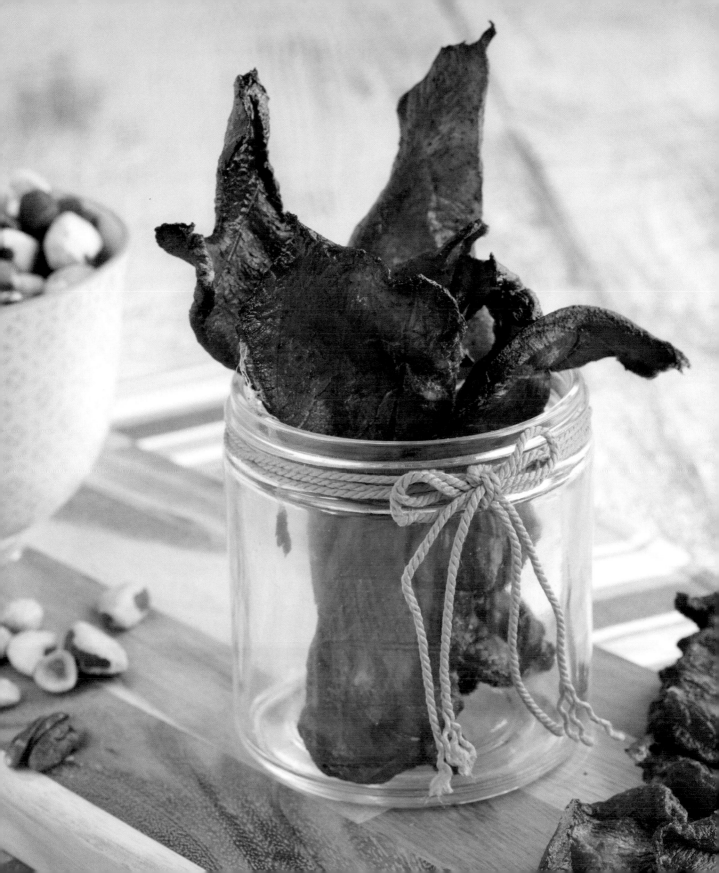

kombucha gelatin

COOK TIME **7 MINS** • CHILL TIME **1 HR** • SERVINGS **4**

NUTS

EGGS

NIGHTSHADES

FODMAPS

SEAFOOD

16 ounces kombucha, divided

4 to 5 tablespoons grass-fed gelatin* (more gelatin means a firmer result)

In a small pot over medium heat, warm 8 ounces of the kombucha until it reaches a simmer, about 5 minutes. Add the gelatin to the pot, slowly at first, and whisk it into the liquid vigorously until all of the gelatin is added. The liquid may become a bit frothy. Whisk and simmer until the gelatin has dissolved, about 2 minutes.

Pour the warm kombucha into a 9-by-11-inch or 9-by-9-inch heat-safe ceramic or glass dish and allow it to cool slightly on your countertop, about 10 to 15 minutes. Gently whisk a few ounces of the cold kombucha into the dish with the gelatin-infused kombucha to slowly reduce the temperature of the warm liquid, then whisk in the remaining cold kombucha. Chill for at least 1 hour, then slice or use a cookie or aspic cutter to create shapes of your choice. Store refrigerated in an airtight container for up to 3 days.

Note: Heating kombucha kills off the beneficial bacteria content of this fermented tea beverage. In fact, heating any raw, fermented food over about 118°F has this effect. Combining the heated kombucha with the chilled kombucha helps retain the probiotic benefit of the cold portion of the drink.

INGREDIENT TIP

*I recommend Great Lakes brand grass-fed gelatin with the orange/red label. Note that the green label variety can be used in smoothies but it doesn't work for this recipe because it will not gel.

CHEF NOTE

You can also make this recipe with brewed herbal tea. Just be sure to brew it extra-strong, with at least 3 bags per 16 ounces of water, and use a flavor with a refreshing taste. ●

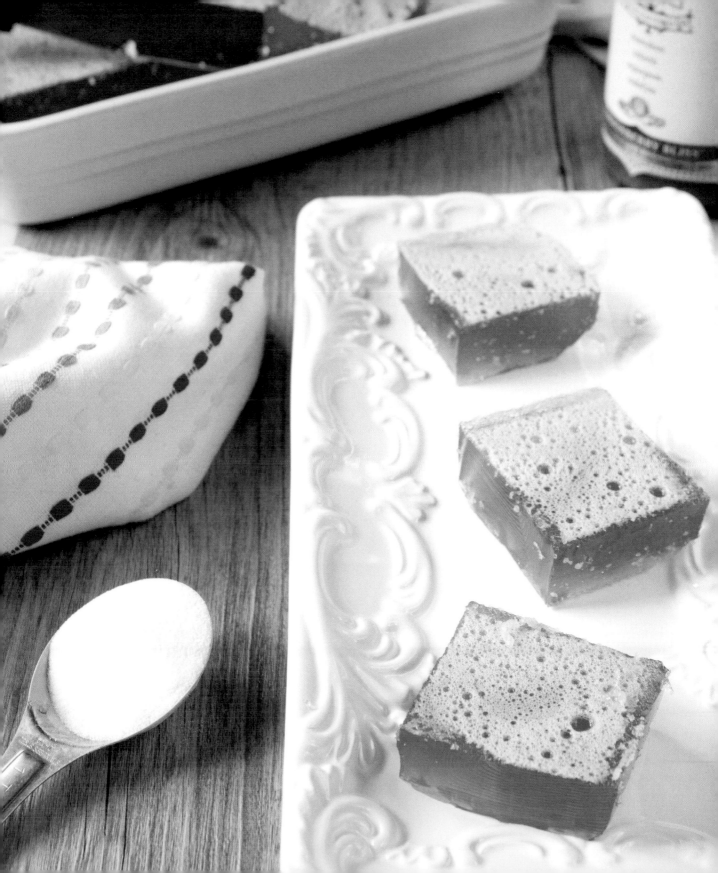

apple spice "granola"

PREP TIME **15 MINS** • COOK TIME **55 MINS** • SERVINGS **12** • YIELD **6 CUPS**

NUTS

EGGS

NIGHTSHADES

FODMAPS

SEAFOOD

2 eggs

1 teaspoon sea salt

2 teaspoons ground cinnamon

1/4 teaspoon ground cloves

2 teaspoons pure vanilla extract

3 green apples, peeled, cored, and roughly chopped

2 cups raw nuts (pecans, almonds, hazelnuts, or a mix)

1/2 cup sunflower seeds

Preheat the oven to 350°F. Line 2 rimmed baking sheets with parchment paper. Note: If you don't have 2 baking sheets, you can bake the granola in 2 batches.

In a large bowl, whisk together the eggs, salt, cinnamon, cloves, and vanilla.

In a food processor, pulse the apples until they achieve the consistency of chunky applesauce, about 5 to 7 times. Place the apples in the middle of a piece of cheesecloth or a clean, thin kitchen towel, pull up the sides of the cheesecloth or towel, and twist it above the apple mixture over the sink to extract as much liquid as possible. Add the apples to the egg mixture and stir to combine.

Add half of the nuts and seeds to the food processor and pulse 8 to 10 times, then add the other half and pulse 8 to 10 times more. The goal is to have some very small pieces and some larger pieces.

Add the nuts into the apple mixture and stir until the nuts are well coated.

Pour the combined mixture onto the prepared baking sheets in a thin layer. (If the layer isn't thin, the mixture won't dry properly; you should be able to see the bottom of the pan in spots.)

Bake for 40 to 45 minutes, carefully flipping the granola after 20 minutes and breaking up the larger pieces. You may also want to rotate your pans at this point if one seems to be browning more than the other.

Once the mixture is browned and the larger pieces are dry to the touch, turn off the oven, leaving the pans in the oven, and prop open the door with a wooden spoon to let any moisture escape. Let the pans sit in the oven for about 10 minutes or until cool.

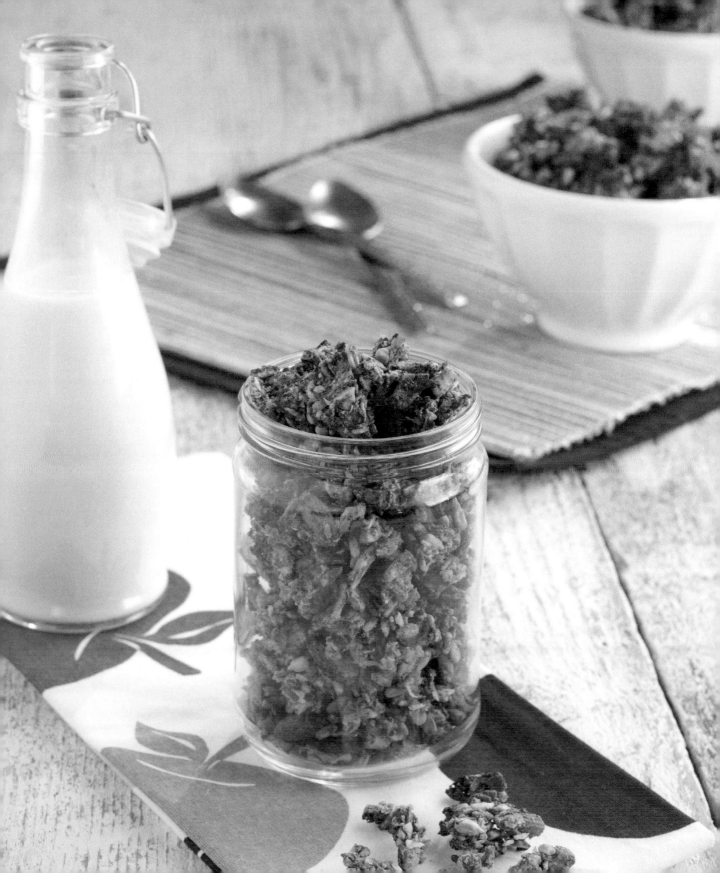

apple chai spice scones

PREP TIME **15 MINS** • COOK TIME **25 MINS** • SERVINGS **8** • YIELD **8 SCONES**

NUTS

EGGS

NIGHTSHADES

FODMAPS

SEAFOOD

SCONES

2 1/2 cups almond flour*

1/2 cup arrowroot flour

2 teaspoons baking powder

1 teaspoon ground cinnamon

1 teaspoon ground cardamom

1/2 teaspoon ground cloves

1/2 teaspoon ground ginger

1/4 teaspoon ground allspice

1/4 teaspoon ground nutmeg

1/2 teaspoon sea salt

1/4 cup butter or ghee, cold

1/4 cup full-fat coconut milk, canned* or homemade (page 210)

2 teaspoons pure vanilla extract

1 egg

2 medium apples, cut into small dice (2 cups)

FROSTING

1/2 cup coconut butter,* melted

1 tablespoon butter, ghee, or coconut oil, chilled and chopped

1 teaspoon pure vanilla extract

2 teaspoons ground cinnamon (optional)

Preheat the oven to 350°F. Line a baking sheet with parchment paper.

In a large bowl, combine the almond flour, arrowroot flour, baking powder, spices, and salt. Cut up the cold butter into 1/4-inch pieces and, using a pastry cutter or a fork, cut it into the flour mixture until individual butter pieces are still visible but the flour mixture takes on a coarse consistency.

In a small bowl, whisk together the coconut milk, vanilla, and egg. Add the coconut milk mixture to the flour mixture, mixing with a fork until it comes together. Add the diced apples and use your hands to knead the dough until it forms a smooth ball.

On a piece of parchment paper, press the dough into a circle about 1-inch thick, evening out the sides with your hands. Cut the circle into 8 wedges. Place the wedges at least 1 inch apart on the prepared baking sheet.

Bake for 20 to 25 minutes or until the edges start to turn golden brown. Remove and let cool to room temperature before frosting.

Make the frosting: In a small bowl, combine the melted coconut butter and butter and stir until the butter is completely melted. Stir in the vanilla. For cinnamon frosting, add the cinnamon and mix thoroughly. The frosting may need to cool slightly to thicken to the desired consistency. Drizzle over the cooled scones and serve.

INGREDIENT TIP
*Check out pages 226–227 for a list of recommended brands.

CHEF NOTE
You can make mini scones by dividing the dough in half before pressing each half into a 1-inch thick circle, slicing it into 8 pieces, and baking for just 15 to 20 minutes. A serving would then be 2 mini scones. ●

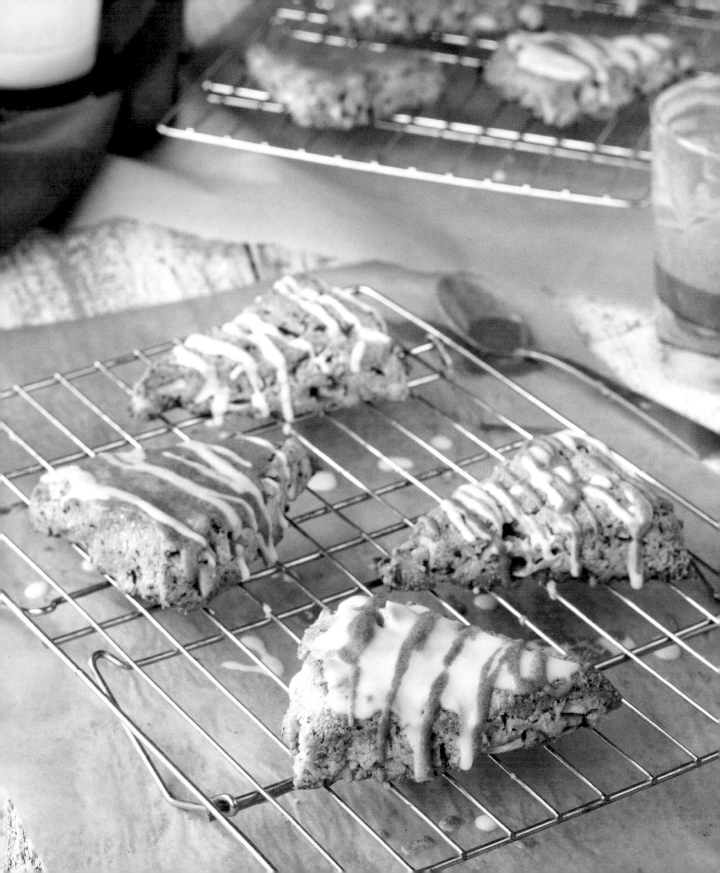

nutty cinnamon crumb cake

PREP TIME **20 MINS** · COOK TIME **30 MINS** · SERVINGS **9**

NUTS

EGGS

NIGHTSHADES

FODMAPS

SEAFOOD

FOR THE BATTER

2 green apples, peeled and cored

3 tablespoons coconut oil or ghee, divided, plus more for greasing the baking dish

2 teaspoons ground cinnamon, divided

dash of ground nutmeg

3 eggs

1 teaspoon pure vanilla extract

1/2 teaspoon apple cider vinegar*

1 cup almond flour*

1/2 teaspoon baking soda

FOR THE TOPPING

1/2 cup pistachios (or other nut of your choice)

1/2 cup almonds (or other nut of your choice)

1 teaspoon ground cinnamon

3 tablespoons coconut oil or ghee

INGREDIENT TIP
*Check out pages 226–227 for a list of recommended brands.

AFTER THE 21DSD
Add 2 tablespoons of maple sugar or maple syrup to the crumb topping mixture before spreading it onto the cake. ●

Preheat the oven to 350°F. Grease a 9-by-9-inch baking dish.

Make the batter: Shred the apples in a food processor or with a box grater. In a pan over medium heat, melt 1 tablespoon of the coconut oil, then add the shredded apples, 1 teaspoon of the cinnamon, and the nutmeg and cook until the apples are slightly browned and soft, approximately 5 minutes. If the apples seem to dry out, add 1 tablespoon of water at a time to help them cook without burning or becoming too dry. Once the apples are cooked, set them in a mixing bowl and place in the freezer for 10 minutes to cool slightly before adding them to the batter.

In a large mixing bowl, whisk the eggs, the remaining 2 tablespoons of coconut oil, vanilla, and vinegar until well combined. Sift the almond flour, baking soda, and remaining 1 teaspoon of cinnamon into the egg mixture and whisk until well combined. Add the cooled apples to the mixture and stir until well incorporated.

Make the topping: Pulse the nuts and cinnamon in a food processor until most of the nuts are finely ground but there are still some slightly larger pieces remaining. Place the nuts in a mixing bowl and add the coconut oil. Mix together until well incorporated, but leave some larger clumps intact.

Pour the batter into the prepared baking dish, then top evenly with the crumb topping. Bake for 30 minutes or until the topping begins to brown and a toothpick comes out clean when inserted into the middle.

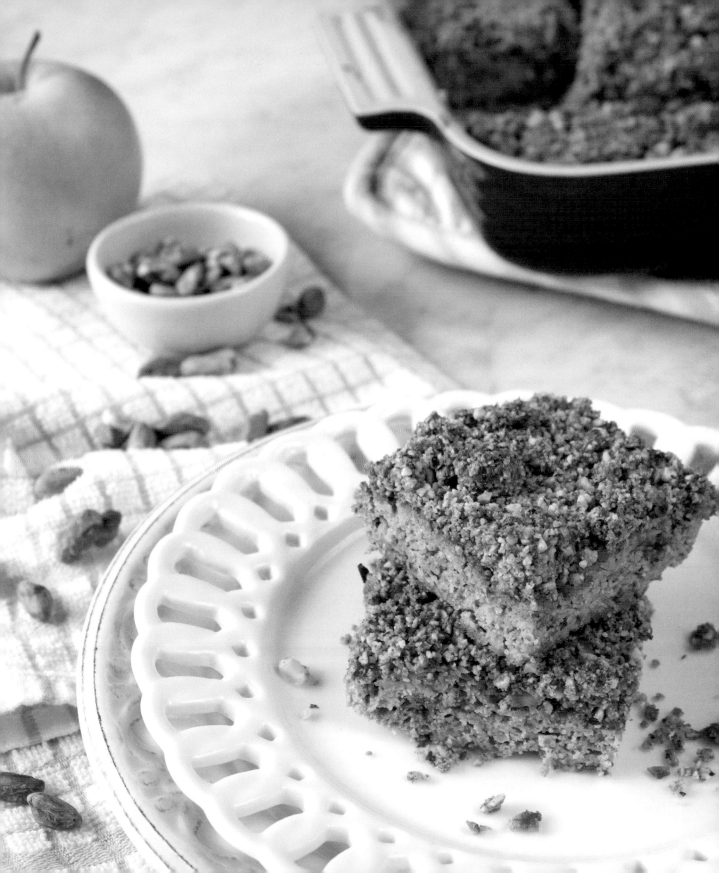

pumpkin spice latte

PREP TIME **5 MINS** • SERVINGS **2**

NUTS

EGGS

NIGHTSHADES

FODMAPS

SEAFOOD

16 ounces hot coffee

1/2 cup full-fat coconut milk, canned* or homemade (page 210), warmed if you prefer

1 to 2 teaspoons pumpkin pie spice

1/2 teaspoon ground cinnamon

2 teaspoons pure vanilla extract

dash of ground nutmeg, for garnish (optional)

INGREDIENT TIP
*Check out pages 226–227 for a list of recommended brands. ●

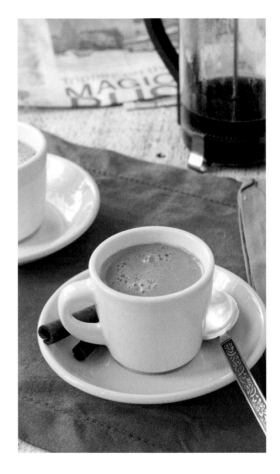

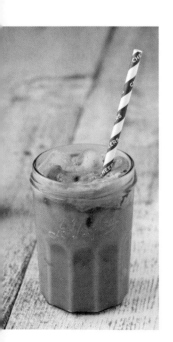

Combine all the ingredients in a blender, starting with 1 teaspoon of the pumpkin pie spice, and blend on high until well incorporated. Taste and add more pumpkin pie spice if desired, and pulse to combine. Serve in coffee cups. Garnish with a dash of nutmeg, if desired.

For an iced version, used chilled coffee and pour over glasses of ice.

sunbutter brownies

PREP TIME **15 MINS** • COOK TIME **35 MINS** • SERVINGS **8** • YIELD **8 BROWNIES**

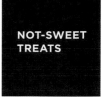

NUTS

EGGS

NIGHTSHADES

FODMAPS

SEAFOOD

coconut oil, for greasing the pan

4 green-tipped bananas

4 eggs

1/2 cup Sunbutter (page 164) or other nut butter

1/2 cup full-fat coconut milk, canned* or homemade (page 210)

1/3 cup unsweetened cocoa powder*

2 teaspoons pure vanilla extract

1/2 teaspoon sea salt

1/4 cup coconut butter, melted (optional)

INGREDIENT TIP
*Check out pages 226–227 for a list of recommended brands. ●

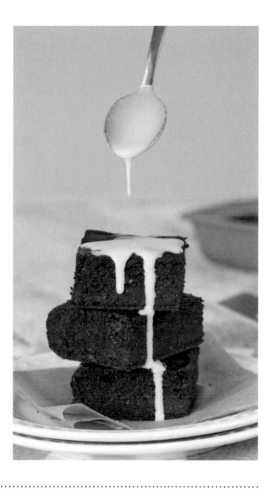

Preheat the oven to 325°F. Grease an 8-by-8-inch baking dish.

In a food processor, mix the bananas, eggs, Sunbutter, and coconut milk until well combined, about 1 minute. Sprinkle in the remaining ingredients and process for another 2 to 3 minutes. Pour the mixture into the prepared baking dish. Bake for 25 to 35 minutes or until the edges are cooked and a toothpick inserted into the middle comes out somewhat wet. (If you bake these until a toothpick comes out clean, they will be overbaked and dry.) Let cool for 10 to 15 minutes before serving.

Drizzle with coconut butter if desired.

banana pecan macaroons
with chocolate glaze

PREP TIME **10 MINS** • COOK TIME **30 MINS** • SERVINGS **8** • YIELD **16 MACAROONS**

NUTS

EGGS

NIGHTSHADES

FODMAPS

SEAFOOD

FOR THE MACAROONS

1 cup pecans

2 green-tipped bananas

2 teaspoons pumpkin pie spice

1 teaspoon ground cinnamon

1/2 teaspoon sea salt

1 teaspoon pure vanilla extract

1/2 teaspoon almond extract

1 1/2 cups unsweetened finely shredded coconut*

FOR THE CHOCOLATE GLAZE

1 tablespoon coconut oil, melted

1 tablespoon butter or ghee, chilled and chopped

2 teaspoons unsweetened cocoa powder*

pinch of sea salt

Preheat the oven to 275°F. Line a baking sheet with parchment paper.

Make the macaroons: Pulse the pecans in a food processor until they have the consistency of a fine nut flour, 20 to 30 seconds. Transfer the pecan flour to a medium mixing bowl and set aside. Place the bananas in the food processor and process for 30 to 45 seconds or until smooth. Add the pumpkin pie spice, cinnamon, salt, vanilla, and almond extract and process for 10 seconds or until well combined.

Transfer the banana mixture to the bowl with the pecan flour and mix well with a spoon. Add the shredded coconut and mix to fully incorporate.

Firmly pack the mixture into a rounded tablespoon or small scoop and tap to release onto the prepared baking sheet. Repeat this process with the remaining mixture. Bake for 25 to 30 minutes or until the edges are golden brown. Allow the macaroons to cool before glazing.

Make the glaze: In a small bowl, combine the melted coconut oil and chopped butter and stir until the butter is completely melted. Stir in the cocoa powder and salt. Drizzle over the macaroons.

INGREDIENT TIP
*Check out pages 226–227 for a list of recommended brands. ●

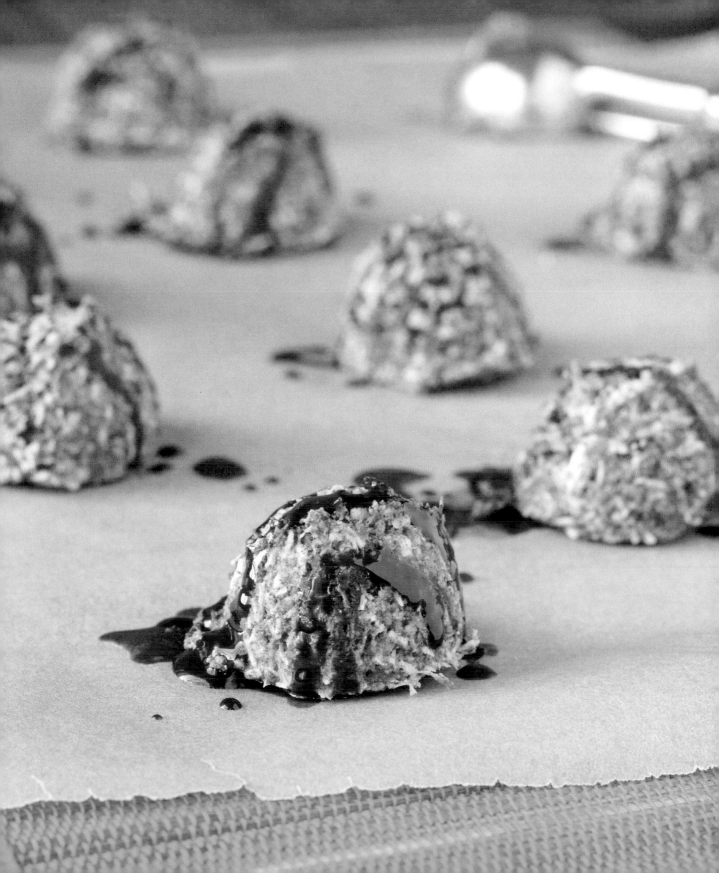

banana-nut cake mini donuts

PREP TIME **10 MINS** • COOK TIME **15 TO 30 MINS** • SERVINGS **6 (1 REGULAR OR 3 MINI DONUTS)**

• YIELD **6 REGULAR OR 18 MINI DONUTS**

NUTS

EGGS

NIGHTSHADES

FODMAPS

SEAFOOD

2 green-tipped bananas, mashed (1/2 cup)

2 eggs

1 teaspoon pure vanilla extract

1 teaspoon hazelnut or almond extract

1/4 cup plus 2 tablespoons full-fat coconut milk, canned* or homemade (page 210)

1/2 teaspoon apple cider vinegar*

1/4 cup coconut flour*

1/2 cup hazelnut flour (or almond flour*)

1/2 teaspoon baking soda

2 teaspoons ground cinnamon

2 tablespoons ghee or coconut oil for greasing the pan

TOPPINGS

2 tablespoons coconut butter,* softened

2 tablespoons almond butter,* softened

2 to 4 tablespoons crushed pecans, hazelnuts, or almonds (optional)

If you're using a donut pan, preheat the oven to 350°F; if you're using an electric mini-donut maker, plug it in to preheat.

In a mixing bowl, whisk together the bananas, eggs, vanilla, hazelnut extract, coconut milk, and vinegar. Sift in the dry ingredients and continue to whisk to combine. Alternatively, for a smoother consistency than whisking by hand allows, you can combine all the ingredients in a food processor or high-speed blender.

Put the batter in a plastic zip-top bag and snip off a small corner (or use a pastry bag). Grease the pan right before filling. Pipe the batter to fill each slot approximately half-full, as the donuts will rise when baking.

If using a donut pan: Bake for 30 minutes or until golden brown.

If using an electric mini-donut maker (as pictured): Cook for 3 to 4 minutes, then repeat until all of the batter is used up (about 3 rounds). Re-grease the donut maker before each round.

Allow the donuts to cool before dipping them in the softened coconut or almond butter (or you may drizzle the butters on top). Sprinkle on the crushed nuts, if desired.

INGREDIENT TIP

*Check out pages 226–227 for a list of recommended brands.

EQUIPMENT TIP

This recipe requires a 6-slot standard donut pan or an electric mini-donut maker (with slots for 7 mini donuts). ●

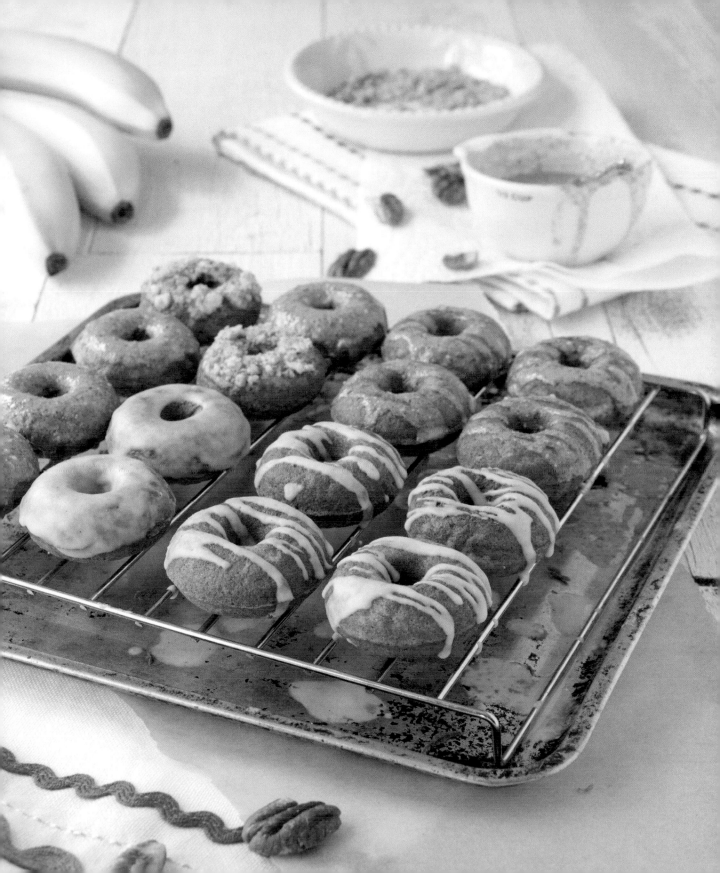

pumpkin spice donuts

PREP TIME **10 MINS** • COOK TIME **15 TO 30 MINS** • SERVINGS **6 (1 REGULAR OR 3 MINI DONUTS)**
• YIELD **6 REGULAR OR 18 MINI DONUTS**

NUTS

EGGS

NIGHTSHADES

FODMAPS

SEAFOOD

1 green-tipped banana, mashed (1/4 cup)

1/4 cup canned pumpkin

2 eggs

1 1/2 teaspoon pure vanilla extract

1/4 cup plus 2 tablespoons full-fat coconut milk, canned* or homemade (page 210)

1/2 teaspoon apple cider vinegar*

1/4 cup coconut flour*

1/2 cup almond flour*

1/2 teaspoon baking soda

1 tablespoon pumpkin pie spice

2 teaspoons ground cinnamon

2 tablespoons ghee to grease the pan

TOPPING OPTIONS

2 tablespoons unsweetened shredded coconut

2 tablespoons almond meal or other crushed nuts

If you're using a donut pan, preheat the oven to 350°F; if you're using an electric mini-donut maker, plug it in to preheat.

In a mixing bowl, whisk the banana, pumpkin, eggs, vanilla, coconut milk, and vinegar together. Sift in the dry ingredients and continue to whisk to combine. Alternatively, for a smoother consistency than whisking by hand allows, you can combine all ingredients in a food processor or high-speed blender.

Put the batter in a plastic zip-top bag and snip off a small corner (or use a pastry bag). Grease the pan right before filling each slot. Pipe the batter to fill the donut pans approximately half-full, as the donuts will rise when baking. Add toppings to the donuts before baking.

If using a donut pan (as pictured): Bake for 30 minutes or until golden brown.

If using a mini-donut maker: Cook for 3 to 4 minutes, then repeat until all of the batter is used up (about 3 batches). Re-grease the donut maker before each round.

INGREDIENT TIP
*Check out pages 226–227 for a list of recommended brands.

EQUIPMENT TIP
This recipe requires a 6-slot standard donut pan or an electric mini-donut maker (with slots for 7 mini donuts). ●

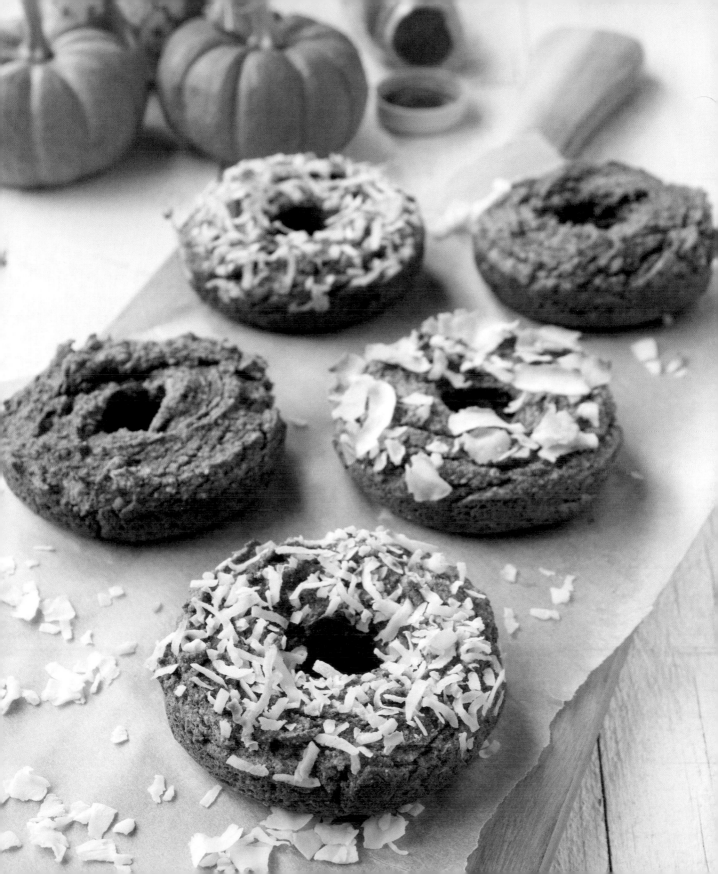

sunbutter truffles
(cocoa-espresso & almond-cocoa nib)

PREP TIME **10 MINS** • YIELD **12 TRUFFLES**

NUTS

EGGS

NIGHTSHADES

FODMAPS

SEAFOOD

FOR THE TRUFFLE BASE

1/3 cup Sunbutter (page 164) or other nut butter,* softened

1/4 cup coconut butter,* softened

FOR COCOA-ESPRESSO TRUFFLES

1 tablespoon finely ground coffee beans

2 tablespoons unsweetened cocoa powder*

1 teaspoon pure vanilla extract

1/3 cup pecans, finely chopped

FOR ALMOND-COCOA NIB TRUFFLES

1 teaspoon almond extract

1 tablespoon cocoa nibs

1/3 cup unsweetened finely shredded coconut

Make the truffle base: Combine the Sunbutter and coconut butter in a small bowl.

Flavor the base: To the base, add the rest of the ingredients for the desired flavor except for the pecans (for the Cocoa-Espresso truffles) or coconut (for the Almond–Cocoa Nib truffles).

Place the bowl in the freezer for 2 to 3 minutes until the mixture is slightly hardened. Scrape out about 2 teaspoons of truffle mixture and roll between your hands into a ball. Roll and press into either the coconut or pecans. Refrigerate to harden before serving, and store any uneaten truffles in the refrigerator for up to a week.

CHEF NOTE
The base for this recipe will suffice for one flavor, not both. To make both flavors, simply double the base recipe, then divide it in half before adding the flavorings.

INGREDIENT TIP
*Check out pages 226–227 for a list of recommended brands. ●

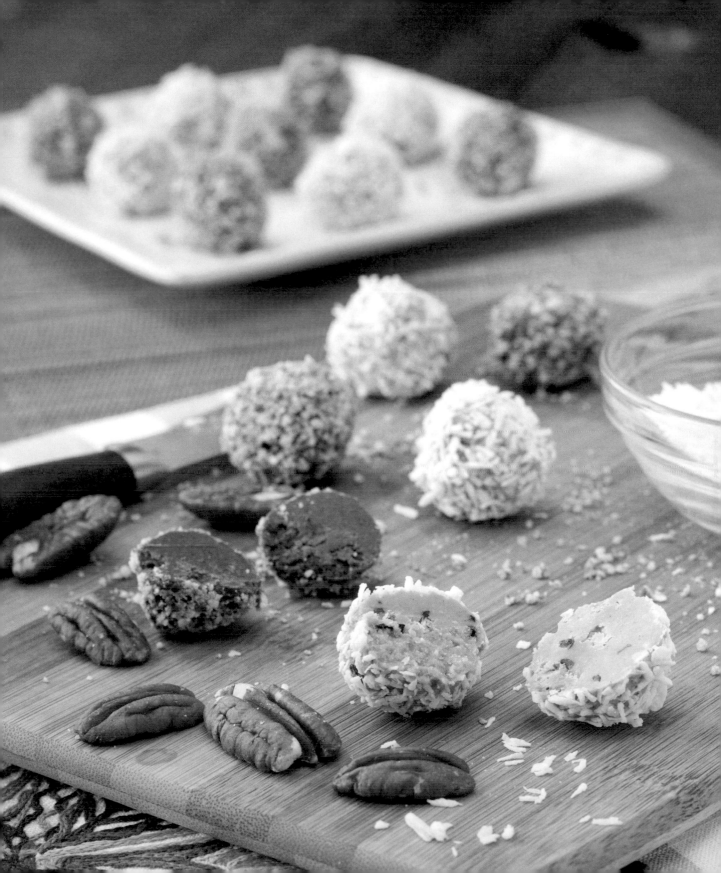

tart lemon torte

PREP TIME **20 MINS** • COOK TIME **25 TO 35 MINS** • SERVINGS **8**

NUTS

EGGS

NIGHTSHADES

FODMAPS

SEAFOOD

CRUST

1 cup almond meal*

1 cup unsweetened
   shredded coconut*

1/4 teaspoon baking soda

1/4 teaspoon sea salt

1 egg

3 tablespoons coconut
   butter,* melted

1 teaspoon pure vanilla
   extract

FILLING

4 green apples, peeled
   and roughly chopped
   (approximately 6 cups)

1 cup lemon juice
   (approximately 7
   lemons)

2 tablespoons lemon zest

4 eggs

1/4 teaspoon sea salt

2 tablespoons coconut
   flour*

Preheat the oven to 350°F.

Make the crust: Combine the almond meal, shredded coconut, baking soda, and salt in a food processor and pulse to combine. Add the egg, coconut butter, and vanilla and process for 1 to 2 minutes or until a dough develops. Press into a 9-inch pie dish or an 8-by-8-inch baking dish. Bake for 10 to 15 minutes or until the crust is golden brown. Remove from the oven; do not turn the oven off.

Make the filling: Combine the apples, lemon juice, lemon zest, eggs, and salt in a food processor or blender and blend until completely combined, about 3 to 5 minutes. Add the coconut flour and process for another 1 to 2 minutes. Pour the filling over the cooked crust and return to the oven. Bake for 15 to 20 minutes or until the edges are golden brown and the center is set. Remove from the oven and let cool to room temperature, then place in the refrigerator to chill completely before serving.

INGREDIENT TIP
*Check out pages 226–227 for a list of recommended brands. ●

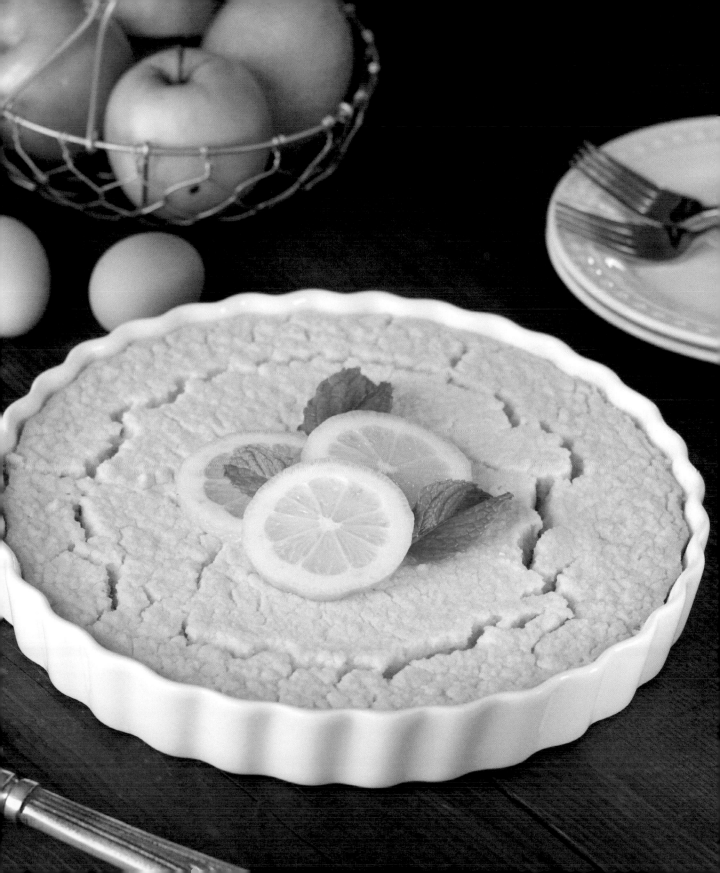

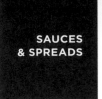

SAUCES & SPREADS

garlic chili paste

PREP TIME **10 MINS** • COOK TIME **10 MINS** • YIELD **1 CUP**

NUTS
EGGS
NIGHTSHADES
FODMAPS
SEAFOOD

10 ounces hot chili peppers (such as serranos, jalapeños, or Thai red chilies), roughly chopped

6 cloves garlic

1 green apple, peeled and chopped

2 tablespoons apple cider vinegar*

1/2 teaspoon sea salt

Combine all the ingredients in a food processor and pulse until you have an even, coarse texture. Put the chili mixture in a small saucepan and cook over medium-high heat for about 10 minutes or until the mixture no longer looks raw and the chilies have released some liquid. Place in an airtight container and keep in the refrigerator for up to 2 weeks.

INGREDIENT TIP
*Check out pages 226–227 for a list of recommended brands. ●

avocado crema

PREP TIME **10 MINS** • YIELD **3/4 CUP**

NUTS
EGGS
NIGHTSHADES
FODMAPS
SEAFOOD

1 avocado

1/2 cup full-fat coconut milk, canned* or homemade (page 210)

1/2 teaspoon ground cumin

1/4 teaspoon sea salt

juice of 1/4 lime

1/8 teaspoon cayenne pepper (optional, omit for nightshade free)

Purée all the ingredients in a food processor or blender until well combined and smooth. The crema will keep for a couple of days when refrigerated in an airtight container.

INGREDIENT TIP
*Check out pages 226–227 for a list of recommended brands. ●

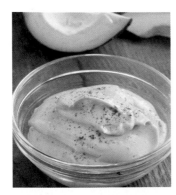

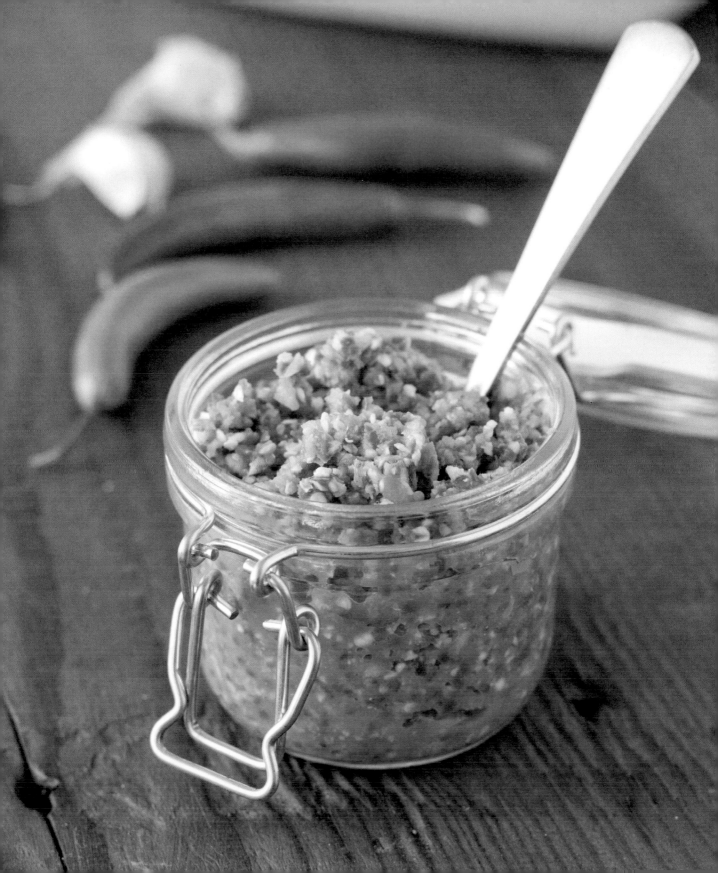

NUTS

EGGS

NIGHTSHADES

FODMAPS

SEAFOOD

creamy cilantro garlic sauce

PREP TIME **10 MINS** • YIELD **1 CUP**

1 cup full-fat coconut milk,
   canned* or homemade
   (page 210)
3 cloves garlic, peeled
1 cup packed fresh cilantro
1/2 teaspoon sea salt

INGREDIENT TIP
*Check out pages
226–227 for a list
of recommended
brands. ●

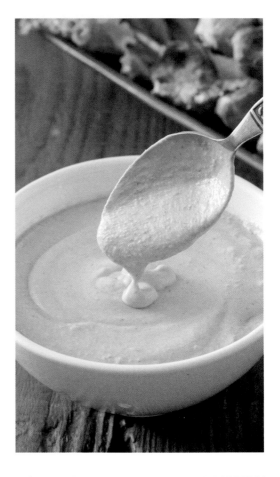

Combine all the ingredients in a blender or food processor and blend until
well combined. Store in a glass jar, refrigerated, for up to 5 days.

bbq sauce

PREP TIME **10 MINS (+KETCHUP AND ONION PREP)** • YIELD **2 CUPS**

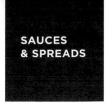

2 cups Sweetener-Free Ketchup (page 216)

1/2 cup Caramelized Onions (page 200)

1/4 cup apple cider vinegar*

1/2 to 1 teaspoon chipotle powder (or less for less heat)**

1 teaspoon mustard powder

1/2 teaspoon paprika

1/2 teaspoon sea salt

1/4 to 1/2 cup water (optional)

NUTS

EGGS

NIGHTSHADES

FODMAPS

SEAFOOD

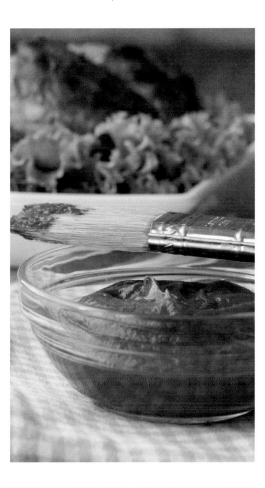

INGREDIENT TIP
*Check out pages 226–227 for a list of recommended brands.

CHEF NOTE
**The newer your chipotle powder is, the hotter it will be! Pepper spices lose their punch as they age, so start with the lesser amount if your batch is new. ●

Combine all the ingredients except the water in a blender and blend on high for 2 to 3 minutes or until well combined. If you prefer a thinner consistency, add the water and blend for another 1 minute. Taste and add more chipotle powder if desired. Store in a glass jar, refrigerated, for up to 5 days.

caramelized onions

PREP TIME **10 MINS** • COOK TIME **45 MINS** • YIELD **ABOUT 1 CUP**

NUTS

EGGS

NIGHTSHADES

FODMAPS

SEAFOOD

2 tablespoon bacon fat, ghee, or coconut oil

4 small onions (yellow, red, or a combination), thinly sliced

1/2 teaspoon sea salt

1/2 teaspoon dried rosemary or thyme (optional)

In a large sauté pan or skillet over medium heat, melt the bacon fat, then place the onions in the pan. Cook the onions for 8 to 10 minutes or until they begin to become translucent, then add the salt and the dried herbs, if using.

Reduce the heat to medium-low and slowly cook the onions, stirring occasionally, allowing them to brown just slightly before stirring each time. If you find that the onions are browning too quickly or are sticking too much, reduce the heat slightly, add 1 to 2 tablespoons of warm water at a time to the pan, and stir it into the onions to keep them cooking evenly. Over the cooking time, the onions will become more and more browned and softened, and eventually they will look as they do in the photo. They will be rich-tasting and richly colored at the end of cooking, around 45 minutes. This process requires low, slow heat; faster, hotter heat will not yield the same results.

CHANGE IT UP
Add 1 to 2 tablespoons of balsamic vinegar to the onions for their last 10 minutes of cooking for a more robust flavor.

CHEF NOTE
Enjoy these onions as a topping for burgers, sausages, or grass-fed hot dogs or mixed into meatloaf, omelets, or the Worth-the-Wait Crustless Quiche (page 54). ●

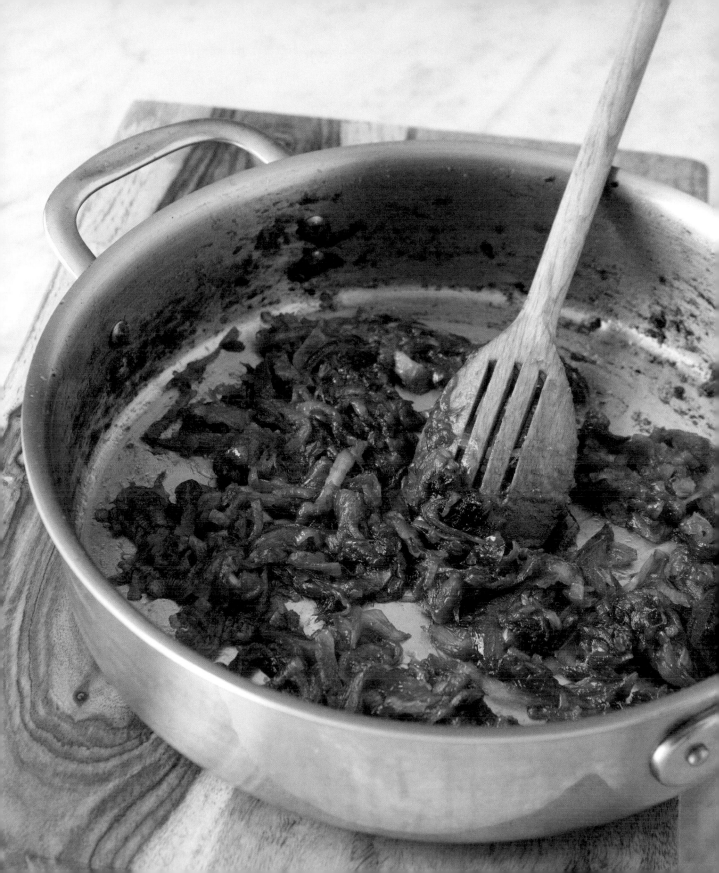

no-honey mustard sauce

PREP TIME **15 MINS** • COOK TIME **20 MINS (+ 1 HR TO CHILL)**
• SERVINGS **8 (1/4 CUP EACH)** • YIELD **2 CUPS**

NUTS

EGGS

NIGHTSHADES

FODMAPS

SEAFOOD

4 green apples, peeled and roughly diced (4 cups)

1 recipe Healthy Homemade Mayonnaise (page 219)

3 tablespoons gluten-free Dijon mustard*

3/4 teaspoon sea salt

1/4 teaspoon black pepper

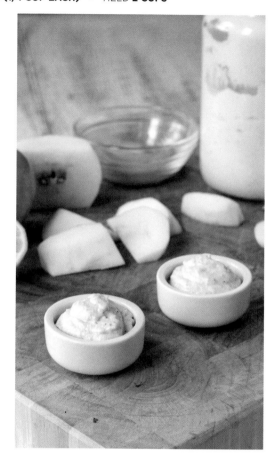

INGREDIENT TIP
*Check out pages 226–227 for a list of recommended brands. ●

Purée the diced apples in a food processor, scraping down the sides often, for about 1 minute or until smooth. Pour the puréed apples into a saucepan and cook over medium heat for 15 to 20 minutes, stirring frequently, until as much liquid as possible is cooked out and the apples are the consistency of a thick paste. Transfer the paste to a bowl and set it in the refrigerator, uncovered, to chill completely, about 1 hour.

Remove the apple paste from the refrigerator and add the remaining ingredients, stirring to completely incorporate. Check for seasoning and add additional salt and pepper if needed. Store in a glass jar, refrigerated, for up to 5 days.

spiced buttery apple spread

PREP TIME **10 MINS** • COOK TIME **20 MINS** • SERVINGS **8 (3 TABLESPOONS EACH)**
• YIELD **1 1/2 CUPS**

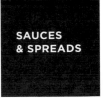

4 green apples, peeled and diced (about 4 cups)

3/4 cup unsalted butter, softened

2 teaspoons ground cinnamon

1/2 teaspoon ground nutmeg

1/4 teaspoon ground cloves

NUTS

EGGS

NIGHTSHADES

FODMAPS

SEAFOOD

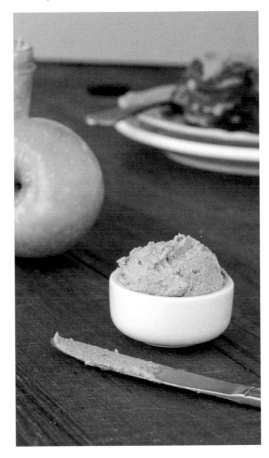

CHEF NOTE
If you don't want to use butter, you can make this spread with ghee or even coconut butter. ●

Purée the chopped apples in a food processor or blender, scraping down the sides often, for about 45 to 60 seconds or until smooth. Pour the puréed apples into a saucepan and cook over medium heat for 15 to 20 minutes, stirring often, until as much liquid as possible is cooked out and the apples are the consistency of a thick paste. Put the paste in a mixing bowl and let cool until it is just warm.

Add the rest of the ingredients to the bowl and mix until well combined. Store in the refrigerator in a glass jar for up to 2 weeks.

thousand island dressing

PREP TIME **5 MINS** · SERVINGS **4** · YIELD **1/2 CUP**

NUTS
EGGS
NIGHTSHADES
FODMAPS
SEAFOOD

1/2 cup Healthy Homemade Mayonnaise (page 219)

1/4 cup Sweetener-Free Ketchup (page 216)

1/4 cup minced dill pickles*

sea salt and black pepper to taste

In a small bowl, whisk together all the ingredients. This dressing should keep well for up to a week in the refrigerator in a glass jar.

apple cider vinaigrette

PREP TIME **5 MINS** · YIELD **ABOUT 3/4 CUP (ABOUT 6 SERVINGS)**

NUTS
EGGS
NIGHTSHADES
FODMAPS
SEAFOOD

1/2 cup extra-virgin olive oil

1/4 cup apple cider vinegar*

1 teaspoon gluten-free Dijon mustard*

1 teaspoon onion powder

sea salt and black pepper to taste

In a small bowl, whisk together all the ingredients. This dressing should keep well for up to a week in the refrigerator in a glass jar.

creamy ranch dressing

PREP TIME **5 MINS** · SERVINGS **4** · YIELD **1/2 CUP**

NUTS
EGGS
NIGHTSHADES
FODMAPS
SEAFOOD

1/4 cup Healthy Homemade Mayonnaise (page 219)

1/4 cup full-fat coconut milk, canned* or homemade (page 210)

1 tablespoon minced fresh dill

2 tablespoons minced fresh chives

1 clove garlic, minced

1 to 2 tablespoons apple cider vinegar* to taste

sea salt and black pepper to taste

In a small bowl, whisk together all the ingredients. Add just 1 tablespoon of the vinegar at first, taste, and add more if needed. This dressing should keep well for up to a week in the refrigerator in a glass jar.

INGREDIENT TIP
*Check out pages 226–227 for a list of recommended brands. ●

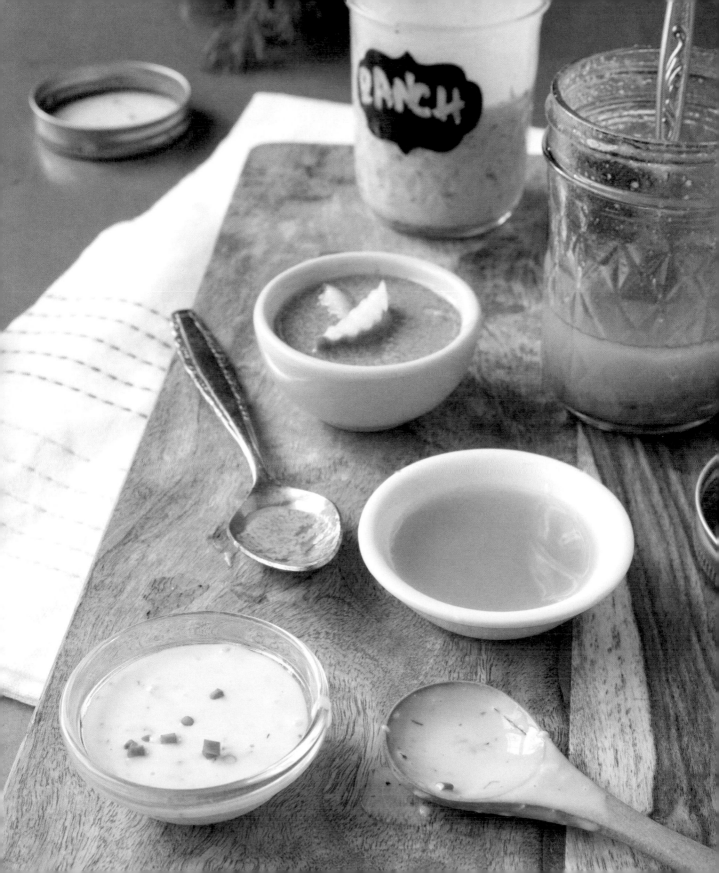

creamy pesto dressing

PREP TIME **5 MINS** • SERVINGS **8** • YIELD **1 CUP**

NUTS

EGGS

NIGHTSHADES

FODMAPS

SEAFOOD

1/2 cup full-fat coconut milk, canned* or homemade (page 210)

1/2 cup Healthy Homemade Mayonnaise (page 219)

1/4 cup Spinach & Walnut Pesto (page 207)

sea salt

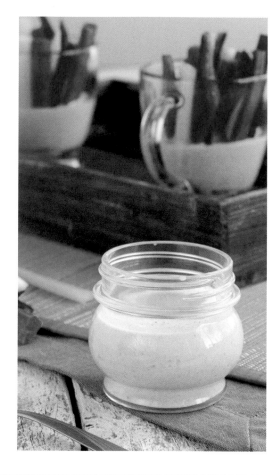

INGREDIENT TIP
*Check out pages 226–227 for a list of recommended brands. ●

In a small bowl, combine all the ingredients and mix well. Add salt to taste. For best flavor, refrigerate for at least 1 hour before serving. Store in a glass jar, refrigerated, for up to 5 days.

spinach & walnut pesto

PREP TIME **15 MINS** • SERVINGS **8** • YIELD **1 CUP**

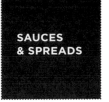

1 cup walnuts
6 cloves garlic
1 teaspoon sea salt
1 cup extra-virgin olive oil
2 cups packed fresh basil
2 cups packed spinach leaves
juice of 1/2 lemon

NUTS

EGGS

NIGHTSHADES

FODMAPS

SEAFOOD

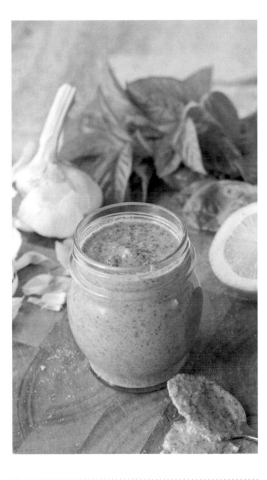

CHEF NOTE
To give this pesto a
different flavor, use
cilantro instead of
basil and pine nuts,
pistachios, or sunflower
seeds in place of the
walnuts. ●

Pulse the walnuts, garlic, salt, and olive oil in a food processor for 2 minutes or until well combined. Add the basil, spinach, and lemon juice and process for an additional 3 to 5 minutes or until the mixture is smooth. Store in a glass jar, refrigerated, for up to 2 weeks.

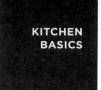

KITCHEN BASICS

bone broth

PREP TIME **5 MINS** • COOK TIME **8 TO 24 HRS** • YIELD **ABOUT 2 1/2 QTS**

NUTS
EGGS
NIGHTSHADES
FODMAPS
SEAFOOD

4 quarts filtered water

1 1/2 to 2 pounds bones (beef knuckle bones, marrow bones, meaty bones, chicken or turkey necks, chicken or turkey carcass bones, or any bones you have on hand)

2 tablespoons apple cider vinegar*

2 teaspoons sea salt

1 head garlic (about 12 cloves), peeled and smashed (optional)

Place all the ingredients in a 6-quart slow cooker. Turn the heat to high and bring the water to a boil. Then reduce the heat to low and cook the broth to cook for a minimum of 8 hours and up to 24 hours. The longer it cooks, the better.

Turn off the slow cooker and allow the broth to cool to room temperature. Strain the broth through a fine-mesh strainer or a colander lined with cheesecloth. Store the broth in glass jars in the refrigerator for up to a week, or freeze for later use.

Before using the broth, chip away at the top and discard any fat that has solidified. You can drink the broth or use it as a base for soups, stews, or any recipe that calls for stock or broth.

INGREDIENT TIP
*Check out pages 226–227 for a list of recommended brands.

FODMAP FREE?
Omit the garlic. ●

vegetable broth

PREP TIME **15 MINS** • COOK TIME **4 TO 8 HRS** • YIELD **ABOUT 2 1/2 QUARTS**

NUTS
EGGS
NIGHTSHADES
FODMAPS
SEAFOOD

1 large onion, chopped

4 large carrots, chopped

4 large celery stalks, chopped

8 cloves garlic, smashed

2 bay leaves

6 to 8 sprigs fresh parsley and/or thyme (optional)

2 teaspoons sea salt

4 quarts filtered water

Place all the ingredients in a 6-quart slow cooker. Turn the heat to high and bring the water to a boil. Then reduce the heat to low and cook the broth for a minimum of 4 hours and a maximum of 8 hours. The longer it cooks, the more flavorful it will become.

Turn off the slow cooker and allow the broth to cool to room temperature. Strain the broth through a fine-mesh strainer or a colander lined with cheesecloth. Place in glass jars and store in the refrigerator for up to a week, or freeze for later use.

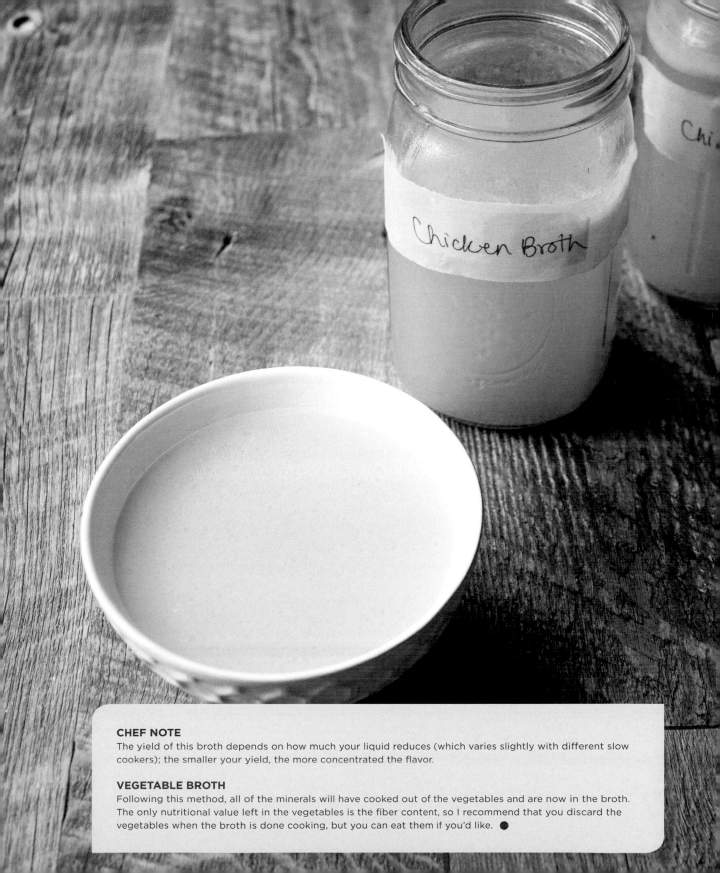

CHEF NOTE
The yield of this broth depends on how much your liquid reduces (which varies slightly with different slow cookers); the smaller your yield, the more concentrated the flavor.

VEGETABLE BROTH
Following this method, all of the minerals will have cooked out of the vegetables and are now in the broth. The only nutritional value left in the vegetables is the fiber content, so I recommend that you discard the vegetables when the broth is done cooking, but you can eat them if you'd like. ●

coconut milk

SOAK TIME **30 MINS** • PREP TIME **10 MINS** • YIELD **4 CUPS**

NUTS

EGGS

NIGHTSHADES

FODMAPS

SEAFOOD

2 cups unsweetened coconut flakes*

4 cups water, divided

1 teaspoon pure vanilla extract

In a medium bowl, combine the coconut flakes and 2 cups of warm (not hot) water. Let sit for at least 30 minutes to soften the coconut flakes.

Put the coconut flakes and soaking water in a blender and add 2 more cups of water. Blend on high for about 1 minute or until the coconut seems fully blended into the water.

If you have a nut milk bag, pour the contents of your blender into the bag and squeeze out all the milk over a large bowl. Transfer the milk to a resealable glass container, add the vanilla, and stir to combine. If you don't have a nut milk bag, use a fine-mesh strainer to strain the milk, pushing the solids against the sides to get as much liquid out as possible. Store the milk in an airtight glass container in the refrigerator for up to 5 days.

You may reserve the leftover solids to add healthy fats and nutrients to smoothies or to make coconut flour.

To make coconut flour: Preheat the oven to 200°F. Spread out the coconut solids in an even layer on a baking sheet, breaking up the larger pieces. Turn off the oven and place the baking sheet in the oven overnight to dry. Place the dehydrated coconut in a food processor and process for approximately 1 to 2 minutes or until finely ground. Try this flour as a replacement for the almond flour in the Chicken Strips (page 78).

INGREDIENT TIP
*Check out pages 226–227 for a list of recommended brands.

EQUIPMENT TIP
A nut milk bag is made of fine mesh cloth and is designed expressly for the purpose of making this type of milk. Visit balancedbites.com/21DSD for recommended brands.

KITCHEN TIP
This recipe works best with a powerful, high-speed blender like a Blendtec or Vitamix. ●

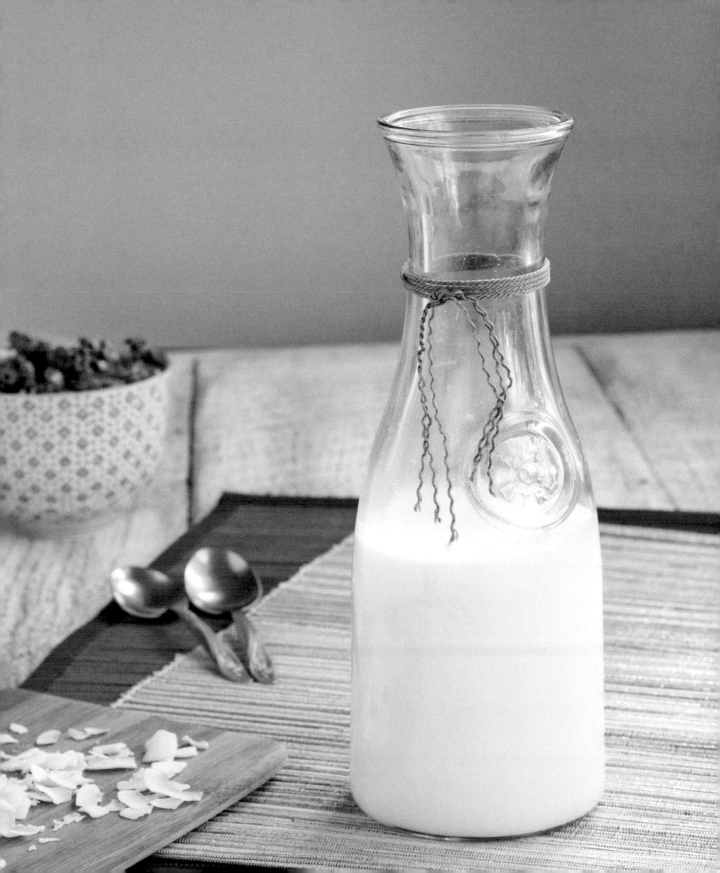

almond milk & meal

PREP TIME **8 HRS + 10 MINS** • YIELD **2 CUPS**

NUTS

EGGS

NIGHTSHADES

FODMAPS

SEAFOOD

2 cups raw almonds

7 cups water, divided

OPTIONAL FLAVORINGS

1/2 to 1 teaspoon
   pure vanilla extract
   (recommended)

1/2 teaspoon cinnamon

1/2 teaspoon unsweetened
   cocoa powder*

To make almond milk: Place the almonds and 4 cups of the water in a glass or other nonporous container and let them soak, covered, in a dark place for 8 hours or overnight.

Strain and rinse the almonds in clean water.

Place the rinsed almonds in a blender with the remaining 3 cups water and blend on high for 2 minutes. Strain the liquid through a nut milk bag or layered cheesecloth over a bowl to catch the milk. Reserve the strained meal. If using optional flavorings, rinse out the blender, place the milk back in with the flavorings, and pulse to combine.

Store almond milk in the refrigerator for up to 5 days.

To make almond meal: Dehydrate the strained meal in a 170°F to 200°F oven for 3 to 4 hours or until completely dry. Pulse in a food processor to smooth out the clumps, and store in the refrigerator to use when a recipe calls for almond meal.

INGREDIENT TIP
*Check out pages 226–227 for a list of recommended brands.

EQUIPMENT TIP
A nut milk bag is made of fine mesh cloth and is designed expressly for the purpose of making this type of milk. Visit balancedbites.com/21DSD for recommended brands.

KITCHEN TIP
This recipe works best with a powerful, high-speed blender like a Blendtec or Vitamix. ●

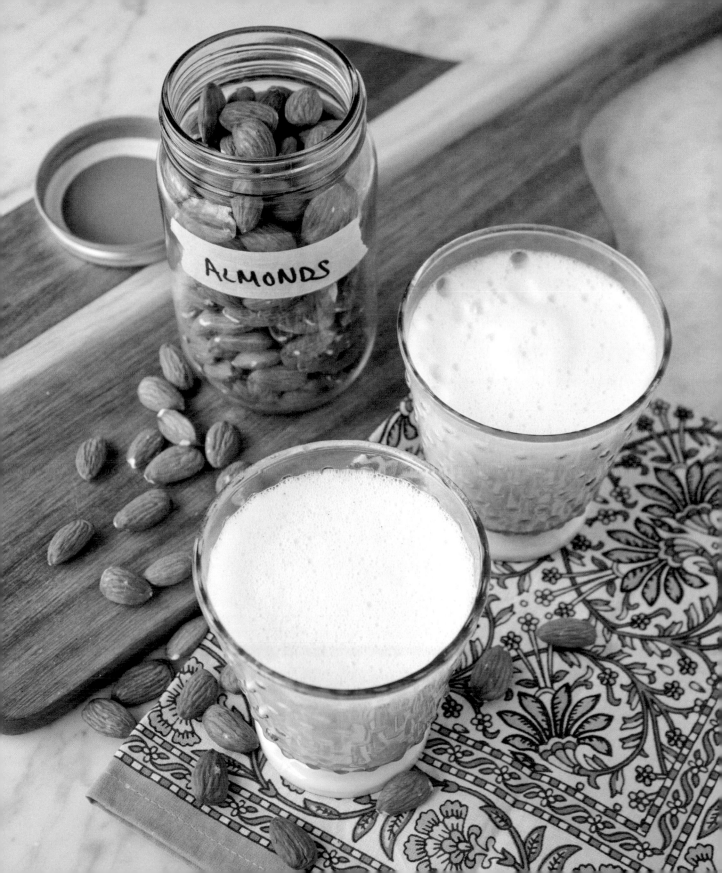

balsamic vinaigrette dressing

PREP TIME **5 MINS** • SERVINGS **8** • YIELD **1 CUP**

NUTS
EGGS
NIGHTSHADES
FODMAPS
SEAFOOD

1/3 cup balsamic vinegar

2/3 cup extra-virgin olive oil

1 teaspoon gluten-free Dijon mustard*

1/2 teaspoon minced shallot or garlic

sea salt and black pepper to taste

1/2 teaspoon dried oregano or basil (optional)

Mix all the ingredients in a resealable glass jar and shake well to combine.

Label and store in the refrigerator for up to a month.

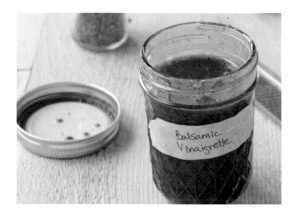

lemon-herb dressing

PREP TIME **5 MINS** • SERVINGS **8** • YIELD **1 CUP**

NUTS
EGGS
NIGHTSHADES
FODMAPS
SEAFOOD

1/3 cup fresh lemon juice

2/3 cup extra-virgin olive oil

1 teaspoon gluten-free Dijon mustard*

1/2 teaspoon minced shallot

sea salt and black pepper to taste

1/2 teaspoon minced fresh cilantro or basil (optional)

Mix all the ingredients in a resealable glass jar and shake well to combine.

Label and store in the refrigerator for up to a month.

INGREDIENT TIP
*Check out pages 226–227 for a list of recommended brands. ●

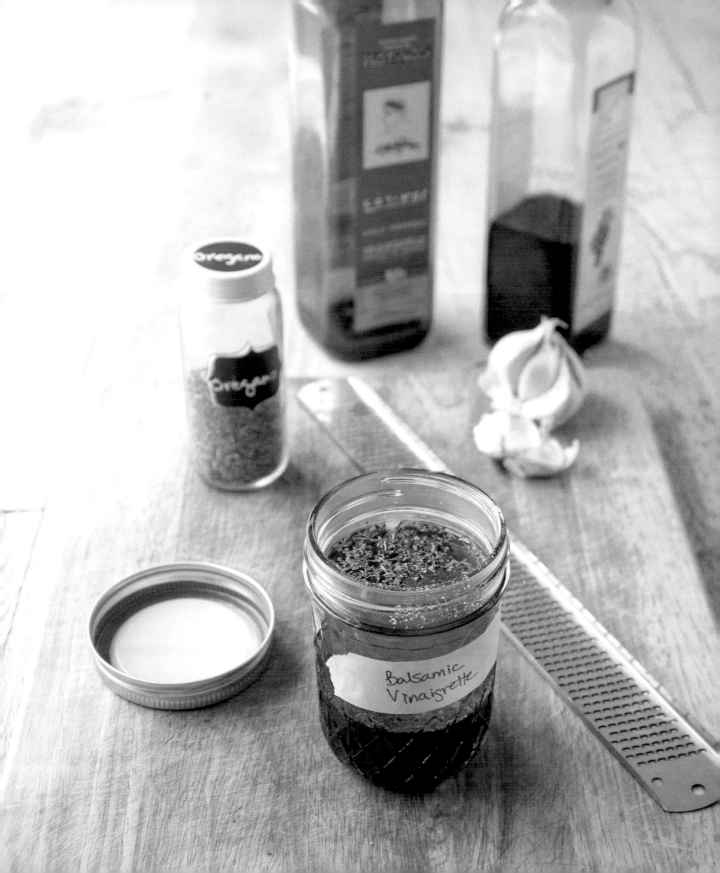

sweetener-free ketchup

PREP TIME **10 MINS** · COOK TIME **4 HRS** · YIELD **16 OUNCES**

1 small onion, diced

2 green apples, peeled and diced

2 cloves garlic, minced

1/2 teaspoon sea salt

1/4 teaspoon allspice

1/4 teaspoon cinnamon

2 pinches of cloves

1/4 teaspoon ground ginger

2 tablespoons apple cider vinegar*

1/4 cup water

1 (6-ounce) can tomato paste

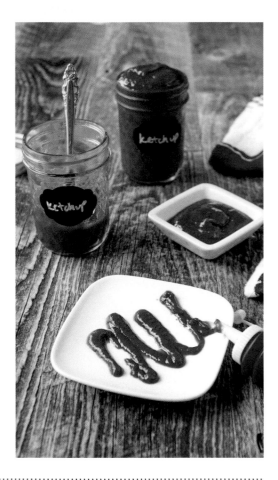

INGREDIENT TIP
*Check out pages 226–227 for a list of recommended brands. ●

Place all the ingredients in a slow cooker and stir to combine. Set the slow cooker to low and cook for 4 hours.

Allow the mixture to cool slightly, then pour into a food processor or high-speed blender and blend until smooth.

Note: When blending or processing warm foods, do not overfill the container, as the heat will cause the contents to expand and they may splatter out.

Once blended, place the ketchup in glass containers and allow it to come to room temperature before refrigerating.

The ketchup should last for several weeks or more in the refrigerator. If you notice a change in color or smell or see any mold growth, toss it and make new batch.

simple marinara

PREP TIME **10 MINS** • COOK TIME **30 MINS** • SERVINGS **4**
• YIELD **ABOUT 24 OUNCES**

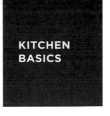

2 tablespoons bacon fat, lard, coconut oil, or other cooking fat*

1/2 cup diced yellow onion

sea salt and black pepper to taste

2 to 3 cloves garlic, grated or minced

1 (28-ounce can) diced tomatoes

1 tablespoon chopped fresh basil

2 tablespoons extra-virgin olive oil, to finish

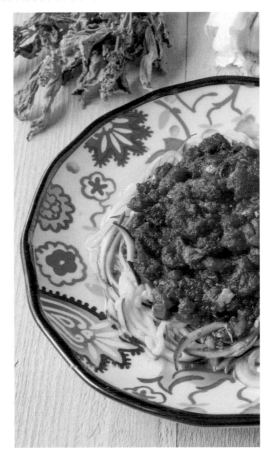

INGREDIENT TIP
*Refer to page 228 to see which fats are best for cooking. ●

NUTS

EGGS

NIGHTSHADES

FODMAPS

SEAFOOD

In a saucepan, melt the cooking fat over medium heat and cook the onion until it is translucent, approximately 5 minutes. Season with salt and pepper.

Add the garlic and cook for an additional 30 seconds. Add the tomatoes, season with additional salt and pepper, and stir to combine. Reduce the heat to low and simmer for 15 to 20 minutes.

Add the basil and simmer for an additional 5 minutes.

Serve over zucchini noodles (pictured). Finish with a drizzle of extra-virgin olive oil for added flavor and richness.

clarified butter & ghee

PREP TIME **5 MINS** • COOK TIME **25 TO 30 MINS (CLARIFIED BUTTER), 35 TO 45 MINS (GHEE)**
• YIELD **25 TO 30 OUNCES**

2 pounds unsalted butter
from pastured cows*

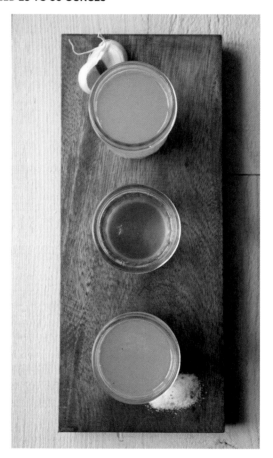

INGREDIENT TIP
*Brands I like include
Kerrygold, SMJÖR,
Organic Pastures, and
Organic Valley Pasture
Butter.

**KEEP IT COOL,
OR DON'T**
Clarified butter and
ghee, when properly
prepared, are shelf
stable. If you didn't
remove all the
milk solids or the
temperature in your
home becomes very
warm, it may go off
sooner than you like.
You can refrigerate
these to make them
last longer. ●

To make clarified butter: Place
the butter in a medium-sized,
heavyweight saucepan and melt it
slowly over low heat. As the butter
comes to a simmer, the milk solids
will float to the top and become
foamy while the separated oil will
become very clear. Skim off the milk
solids and remove the butter from the
heat. Pour it through cheesecloth to
strain out any remaining milk solids,
and store the strained liquid in a
glass jar.

To make ghee: Follow the
instructions for making clarified
butter, but allow the milk solids to
continue to cook slowly until they
become browned and begin to sink
to the bottom of the pan. When there
are no longer any solids waiting to
brown and sink to the bottom of
the oil, the ghee is finished. Pour it
through cheesecloth to strain out the
browned milk solids, and store the
strained liquid in a glass jar.

healthy homemade mayonnaise

PREP TIME **15 MINS** • YIELD **3/4 CUP**

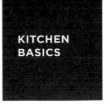

2 egg yolks

1 tablespoon fresh lemon juice

1 teaspoon gluten-free Dijon mustard*

1/2 cup macadamia nut oil or other oil (see page 228)

1/4 cup extra-virgin olive oil

NUTS

EGGS

NIGHTSHADES

FODMAPS

SEAFOOD

INGREDIENT TIP

*Check out pages 226–227 for a list of recommended brands.

KITCHEN TIP

You can also use a handheld immersion blender or a small blender. If using a regular-sized blender, double the recipe to make blending easier. Use the opening at the top of your blender to slowly drizzle in the oil. ●

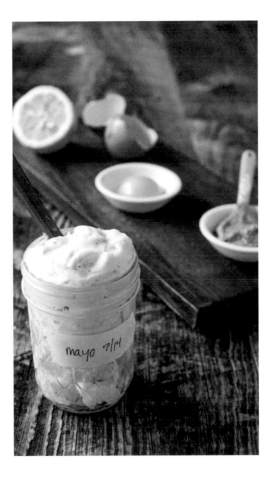

In a medium-sized mixing bowl, whisk together the egg yolks, lemon juice, and mustard until blended and bright yellow, about 30 seconds. Begin adding 1/4 cup of the macadamia nut oil to the yolk mixture a few drops at a time, whisking constantly. Gradually add the remaining 1/4 cup of macadamia nut oil and the olive oil in a slow, thin stream, whisking constantly, until the mayonnaise is thick and lighter in color.

Store in the refrigerator for up to a week.

For all sauces and dressings, combine all the ingredients in a small mixing bowl and whisk together vigorously. Store in a sealed glass jar in the refrigerator for up to a week.

avo-goddess sauce

PREP TIME **5 MINS** • SERVINGS **4** • YIELD **ABOUT 1/2 CUP**

NUTS
EGGS
NIGHTSHADES
FODMAPS
SEAFOOD

1/2 avocado

1/4 cup full-fat coconut milk, canned* or homemade (page 210)

juice of 1/2 lemon

1/2 clove garlic, minced or grated

1 to 2 teaspoons chopped fresh chives

sea salt and black pepper to taste

creamy ginger lime dressing

PREP TIME **5 MINS** • SERVINGS **4** • YIELD **ABOUT 1/2 CUP**

NUTS
EGGS
NIGHTSHADES
FODMAPS
SEAFOOD

1/2 to 1 teaspoon minced fresh ginger

zest and juice of 1/2 lime

1/4 cup full-fat coconut milk, canned* or homemade (page 210)

1/4 cup + 2 tablespoons macadamia nut oil

spicy sesame ginger dressing

PREP TIME **5 MINS** • SERVINGS **4** • YIELD **ABOUT 1/2 CUP**

NUTS
EGGS
NIGHTSHADES
FODMAPS
SEAFOOD

1/4 cup cold-pressed sesame oil

juice of 2 limes

1/2 to 1 teaspoon minced fresh ginger

pinch of red pepper flakes, or to taste

sea salt and black pepper to taste

avo-ziki sauce

PREP TIME **5 MINS** • SERVINGS **4** • YIELD **ABOUT 1/2 CUP**

NUTS
EGGS
NIGHTSHADES
FODMAPS
SEAFOOD

1 avocado

1/4 cup grated cucumber

1 small clove garlic, grated

juice of 1 lemon

2 tablespoons extra-virgin olive oil

sea salt and black pepper to taste

1 teaspoon minced fresh dill

INGREDIENT TIP
*Check out pages 226–227 for a list of recommended brands. ●

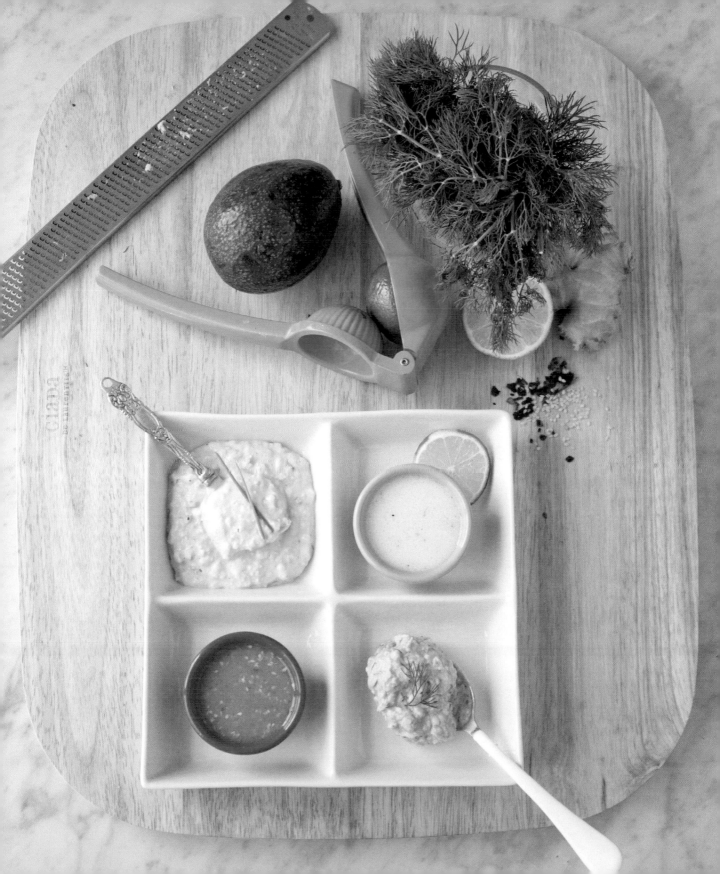

spice blends

Use these blends as they appear in recipes throughout the book—or use them anytime!

SMOKY SPICE BLEND

1 tablespoon chipotle powder
1 tablespoon smoked paprika
1 tablespoon onion powder
1/2 tablespoon ground cinnamon
1 tablespoon sea salt
1/2 tablespoon black pepper

PREP TIME **5 MINS** • YIELD **5 TABLESPOONS**

Combine all the spices in a bowl and store in a small container.

ITALIAN SAUSAGE SPICE BLEND

1 teaspoon sea salt
1 tablespoon ground fennel seeds
1 tablespoon ground sage
1 tablespoon granulated garlic
1 tablespoon onion powder
1/4 teaspoon white pepper (or 1 teaspoon black pepper)
2 teaspoons dried parsley (optional)

PREP TIME **5 MINS** • YIELD **~5 TABLESPOONS**

Combine all the spices in a bowl and store in a small container.

To make sausage, use 2 tablespoons per pound of meat.

CHORIZO SPICE BLEND

2 tablespoons chipotle powder
1 tablespoon smoked paprika
1 tablespoon onion powder
1 tablespoon granulated garlic
1/2 tablespoon sea salt
1 teaspoon black pepper

PREP TIME **5 MINS** • YIELD **~6 TABLESPOONS**

Combine all the spices in a bowl and store in a small container.

Use 2 tablespoons of Chorizo Spice Blend plus 1 tablespoon of apple cider vinegar per pound of meat.

SWEET & SAVORY SPICE BLEND

1 tablespoon granulated garlic
1 tablespoon onion powder
1 tablespoon ground cinnamon
1 tablespoon paprika
1 teaspoon ground cumin
1 tablespoon black pepper
2 teaspoons sea salt

PREP TIME **5 MINS** • YIELD **6 TABLESPOONS**

Combine all the spices in a bowl and store in a small container.

NIGHTSHADE FREE?
Omit the following from your blends: paprika, chili powder, chipotle powder, and red pepper flakes.

FODMAP FREE?
Eliminate the onion powder and granulated garlic. ●

SOUTHWESTERN BLEND

2 tablespoons chili powder
1 tablespoon ground coriander
1 tablespoon sea salt
1 tablespoon dried oregano
1 tablespoon paprika
1 tablespoon ground cumin
1 teaspoon cayenne pepper

PREP TIME **5 MINS** • YIELD **~7 TABLESPOONS**

Combine all the spices in a bowl and store in a small container.

BREAKFAST SAUSAGE BLEND

1 1/2 tablespoons sea salt
1 tablespoon dried sage
1 tablespoon dried thyme
1 tablespoon dried rosemary, chopped
1/2 teaspoon ground nutmeg
1 teaspoon dried parsley
1 teaspoon paprika
1 teaspoon red pepper flakes

PREP TIME **5 MINS** • YIELD **~5 1/2 TABLESPOONS**

Combine all the spices in a bowl and store in a small container.

Use 2 tablespoons per pound of ground pork.

THAI SPICE BLEND

1 tablespoon ground turmeric
1 tablespoon ground coriander
1 tablespoon ground cumin
2 teaspoons granulated garlic
1 teaspoon onion powder
1 teaspoon ground ginger
1 teaspoon sea salt
1 teaspoon black pepper
pinch of red pepper flakes
1 cardamom pod, smashed

PREP TIME **5 MINS** • YIELD **5 TABLESPOONS**

Combine all the spices in a bowl and store in a small container.

GREEK SPICE BLEND

2 tablespoons dried lemon zest
2 tablespoons dried oregano
1 tablespoon granulated garlic
1 teaspoon sea salt
2 teaspoons black pepper

PREP TIME **5 MINS** • YIELD **6 TABLESPOONS**

Combine all the spices in a bowl and store in a small container.

To dry lemon zest before using it in this spice blend, place it on a baking sheet in a 200°F oven for about 1 hour.

INDIAN SPICE BLEND

2 tablespoons onion powder
1 tablespoon garam masala
1 tablespoon ground coriander
1 teaspoon sea salt
1 teaspoon black pepper
1/2 teaspoon ground cinnamon
1/2 teaspoon red pepper flakes

PREP TIME **5 MINS** • YIELD **5 TABLESPOONS**

Combine all the spices in a bowl and store in a small container.

guide to **common food allergens**
(and other potentially irritating but 21DSD-friendly foods)

 If a recipe in this book calls for potentially allergenic ingredients, the category into which those ingredients fall is highlighted in the list that appears in the page's outer margin. If the recipe can be made *without* those ingredients, an ingredient tip or comment will note to omit them or suggest a replacement. For example, a recipe may read "FODMAP FREE? Omit the shallots." If you find that you react to certain foods, I recommend working with a naturopath, chiropractor, or other practitioner who can submit tests to a lab for analysis in order to determine the root cause of the intolerance.

COMMON REACTIONS TO IRRITATING FOODS INCLUDE (BUT ARE NOT LIMITED TO):

Allergic reactions ranging from mild to full anaphylactic shock. Sensitivities can result in headaches, skin reactions (acne, eczema, psoriasis), digestive distress (bloating, gas, irregular bowel movements), or joint pain or stiffness.

TO LEARN MORE ABOUT DIGESTION, HOW IT SHOULD WORK, AND WHAT TO DO WHEN THINGS GO WRONG, CHECK OUT MY BOOK *PRACTICAL PALEO*.

NUTS

ARE **HIGHLIGHTED** IF THE RECIPE CONTAINS:
All nuts (whole, butters, flours, and meals)—almonds, brazil nuts, chestnuts, filberts/hazelnuts, macadamia nuts, pecans, pine nuts, pistachios, or walnuts

BUT **NOT** IF THE RECIPE CONTAINS:
Coconut—Most people who are reactive to nuts do not find that they also react to coconut, although you may have a separate coconut allergy or sensitivity.
Peanuts and cashews—These are not allowed on the program and therefore are never included in the recipes.
Seeds—If you are allergic to nuts (and are not following autoimmune modifications), seeds can typically be substituted 1:1 in recipes.

REPLACEMENTS FOR NUTS:
Seeds and seed flours
Coconut—But note that you cannot substitute coconut flour for nut flours 1:1.

EGGS

ARE **HIGHLIGHTED** IF THE RECIPE CONTAINS:
Whole eggs, egg yolks, egg whites, or mayonnaise

REPLACEMENTS FOR EGGS (NOT RECOMMENDED FOR RECIPES THAT CALL FOR MORE THAN 2 OR 3 EGGS):
Gelatin—Dissolve 1 tablespoon unflavored gelatin in 1 tablespoon cold water, then add 2 tablespoons boiling water and whisk vigorously until frothy.
Flax or chia seeds—Soak 1 tablespoon ground flax or chia seeds in 3 tablespoons water for 15 minutes.
Arrowroot starch—Replace 1 egg with 2 tablespoons arrowroot starch.
Green-tipped banana: Use 1/4 cup (about 1 banana) per egg.

Note: These are suggestions, but I have not tested each of them in the recipes that contain eggs. If you decide to try one in a recipe, please be aware that it may not turn out exactly as it would have if you had used eggs.

Sources: foodsubs.com, mnn.com, stanfordhospital.org

NIGHTSHADES

ARE **HIGHLIGHTED** IF THE RECIPE CONTAINS:
Tomatoes, white potatoes, peppers (bell and hot, including pepper spices like chili powder, cayenne, and chipotle powder), or eggplant

BUT **NOT** IF THE RECIPE CONTAINS:
Black pepper or sweet potatoes, which are not nightshades.

REPLACEMENTS FOR NIGHTSHADES:
For bell peppers and pepper spices—In cooked recipes, I recommend using spices, seasonings, and herbs to enhance the flavor of dishes when peppers are removed. For raw applications or dipping, try carrots, cucumbers, or celery sticks.
For eggplant—Use zucchini, summer squash, or butternut squash.
For tomatoes—For sauces and stews, try canned pumpkin or coconut milk. For salads or salsas, try cucumber or green apples.
For white potatoes—Use cauliflower, butternut or winter squash, or sweet potatoes (if following the Energy Modifications).

FODMAPS

ARE **HIGHLIGHTED** IF THE RECIPE CONTAINS:
Apples, artichokes, avocado, beets, bell peppers, broccoli, Brussels sprouts, cauliflower, cabbage, coconut, eggplant, fennel, garlic, leeks, mushrooms, onions (all kinds), or shallots.

BUT **NOT** IF THE RECIPE CONTAINS:
A lot of foods that are high in FODMAPs are not included on The 21DSD, including many grains, legumes, and fruits. If you are completing The 21DSD on Level 1 and suspect that you are reacting to the grains or beans you are eating, avoid them and see how you feel. There are also some foods that may contain low levels of FODMAPs, like green beans, that are not flagged in recipes.

REPLACEMENTS FOR FODMAPS:
Low or FODMAP-free vegetables including bok choy, carrots, celery, cucumber, leafy greens, summer squash, and tomatoes.
Extra-virgin olive oil—Add to salads or meals instead of avocado to increase the fat.
Nuts or nut milk—Use in place of coconut or coconut milk.

SEAFOOD

IS **HIGHLIGHTED** IF THE RECIPE CONTAINS:
All fish and shellfish; fish sauce

REPLACEMENTS FOR SEAFOOD:
Use other types of protein—Chicken, pork, turkey, or red meats.

MORE DETAILS ON NIGHTSHADES & FODMAPS

Nightshades are a family of plants that contain specific alkaloid compounds that can be irritating to those suffering from joint pain and inflammation.

Note that if a packaged food names "spices" as an ingredient without listing specific ones, paprika is probably among them. People who are sensitive to nightshades should avoid these items because paprika is derived from peppers. Other, less frequently consumed nightshades include tomatillos, goji berries, cape gooseberries (but not normal gooseberries), ground cherries (but not Bing or Rainier cherries), garden huckleberries (but not blueberries), and ashwagandha (an herb), as well as tobacco. If you suffer from joint pain or inflammation, arthritis, cracking, or any other joint-related issues, you may want to eliminate nightshades from your diet for the duration of The 21DSD.

FODMAP is an acronym that stands for "fermentable oligosaccharides, disaccharides, monosaccharides, and polyols." FODMAPs are carbohydrates that can be difficult for some people to digest, resulting in symptoms varying from gas and bloating to diarrhea, constipation, or a combination or alternation of the two. Unlike foods that can't be tolerated as a result of incomplete digestion within the small intestine, FODMAP foods become irritating for the following reasons:

- Overgrowth of the wrong type of bacteria in the system (dysbiosis)
- Overgrowth of bacteria in the wrong part of the digestive system, usually the small intestine, where bacteria don't normally live (a condition known as small intestinal bacterial overgrowth, or SIBO)
- Low stomach acid production or secretion, which also contributes to the previous two bacterial issues
- A gut pathogen or infection often acquired during travel abroad

FRESH**PRODUCTS**

APPLEGATE FARMS MEATS
Most grocery stores
Deli meats, bacon

BUBBIES SAUERKRAUT
Most grocery stores
All flavors approved; when in doubt,
check ingredients

FAB FERMENTS
Online: fabferments.com

G.T.'S SYNERGY
Whole Foods Market, most grocery stores
Kombucha: various flavors

PETE'S PALEO
Online: petespaleo.com
21DSD-approved meals, bacon

REAL PICKLES
*Whole Foods Market, local organic
grocers/co-ops*

TESSEMAE'S ALL NATURAL
*Online: tessemaes.com; Whole Foods
Market*
Dressing/marinade/dip: Balsamic,
Cracked Pepper, Hot Sauce/Wing
Sauce (mild, medium, hot), Oil-
Free Italian, Lemon Chesapeake,
Lemon Garlic, Lemonette, Red Wine
Vinaigrette, Zesty Ranch
Excludes Soy Ginger & Matty's BBQ
(I recommend adding Kasandrinos
Extra Virgin Olive Oil to the oil-free
varieties if you purchase those)

WHOLLY GUACAMOLE
*Online: eatwholly.com; Whole Foods
Market, Trader Joe's (as store brand),
Costco, local organic grocers/co-ops*

WILDBRINE
*Whole Foods Market, local organic
grocers/co-ops*
Sauerkraut: various flavors

21DSD **JERKY**

PALEO JERKY
Online: huntedandgathered.com.au
Note: The sugar content is negligible,
so this jerky is okay for The 21DSD.

SOPHIA'S SURVIVAL FOOD
Online: grassfedjerkychews.com
Beef jerky: Mild and Spicy
*Excludes Chipotle Raisin flavor—which
is fantastic for after your 21DSD!*

STEVE'S ORIGINAL
Online: stevespaleogoods.com
Just Jerky & PaleoStix varieties
*Excludes Berky, Dried Fruit, PaleoKits,
and PaleoKrunch*

US WELLNESS MEATS
Online: bit.ly/USWMBB
Jerky, Pemmican
Excludes Honey & Cherry flavor

FATS&**OILS**

ARTISANA & NUTIVA BRANDS
*Online: artisana.com, Amazon.com; local
grocers*
Coconut oil

FATWORKS
Online: fatworksfoods.com
Duck fat, lard, and tallow

KASANDRINOS OLIVE OIL
Online: kasandrinos.com

KERRYGOLD BUTTER
*Trader Joe's, Costco, Whole Foods
Market, local grocers*

PURE INDIAN FOODS GHEE
*Online: pureindianfoods.com,
Amazon.com; local grocers*

SMJÖR BUTTER
Grocery stores

TROPICAL TRADITIONS
See also: Nuts & Baking Items
Online: tropicaltraditions.com
Coconut oil (I recommend Green Label
for the best taste)

WILDERNESS FAMILY NATURALS
Online: wildernessfamilynaturals.com
Organic coconut oils, natural red palm
oil, sesame seed oil, olive oil, Mary's
Sauté Oil (named after Mary Enig,
author of *Know Your Fats*: blend of
virgin coconut oil, extra-virgin olive oil,
and unrefined sesame seed oil)

SAUCES&**DRESSINGS**
See also: Fresh Products

ANNIE'S & EDEN FOODS
*Online: Amazon.com; Whole Foods
Market, local grocers*
Gluten-free mustards

ARIZONA GUNSLINGER
*Online: azgunslinger.com; selected
retailers*
Organic harvest gluten-free hot sauces

BIONATURAE
*Online: tropicaltraditions.com;
Whole Foods Market*
Balsamic vinegar

BRAGG'S
Local grocers
Organic apple cider vinegar

COCONUT SECRET
*Online: coconutsecret.com, Amazon.
com; Whole Foods Market, local organic
grocers/co-ops*
Coconut aminos, coconut vinegar

FRANKS REDHOT
*Online: franksredhot.com, Amazon.com;
major grocery stores*

RED BOAT FISH SAUCE
*Online: redboatfishsauce.com; Whole
Foods Market, local grocers*

COCONUT, NUTS BUTTERS&FLOURS

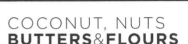

ARTISANA & NUTIVA BRANDS

Online: artisana.com, Amazon.com; local organic grocers/co-ops
Almond butter (roasted or raw), coconut butter, coconut manna—sold in jars and handy travel-sized packets
Excludes cashew, walnut, pecan, and macadamia butters (all are blended with cashews), & Cacao Bliss—which are fantastic for after your 21DSD!

BARNEY BUTTER

Online: barneybutter.com, Amazon.com
Barney Bare only
Excludes smooth, crunchy, and squeeze packs (at this time, the Barney Bare is not available in squeeze packs)

BOB'S RED MILL

Online: bobsredmill.com, Amazon.com; major grocery stores
Almond, coconut, hazelnut meal/flours

HONEYVILLE

Online: honeyville.com
Blanched almond meal/flour

JUSTIN'S NUT BUTTER

Online: justins.com, Amazon.com; local grocers
Original only—sold in jars and handy travel-sized packets
Excludes honey, maple, chocolate, and vanilla almond butters, all peanut butters, and chocolate hazelnut butter

MARANATHA

Online: maranathafoods.com, Amazon.com; Whole Foods Market, organic grocers
Almond butters, sunflower seed butter, sesame tahini

ONCE AGAIN NUT BUTTERS

Online: onceagainnutbutter.com; Whole Foods Market
Almond butter, tahini

PALEO MEENUT BUTTER

Online: meeeatpaleo.com

SUNBUTTER (NUT-FREE)

Online: sunbutter.com, Amazon.com; grocery stores
Only the organic, unsweetened variety

THAI KITCHEN

Online: Amazon.com; grocery stores
Full-fat coconut milk, canned

TRADER JOE'S

traderjoes.com for locations
Sunflower seed butter, almond butter

TROPICAL TRADITIONS

Online: tropicaltraditions.com
Shredded coconut, coconut chips, coconut flour, coconut cream concentrate

WHOLE FOODS STORE BRAND

wholefoodsmarket.com for locations
Full-fat coconut milk

WILDERNESS FAMILY NATURALS

Online: wildernessfamilynaturals.com
Coconut, coconut flour, coconut cream concentrate, almonds, crispy almonds, almond butter

HERBAL TEAS

TRADITIONAL MEDICINALS

Online: Amazon.com; Whole Foods Market, local organic grocers/co-ops
All herbal tea varieties

BAKING ITEMS

IF YOU CARE, PAPER CHEF BRANDS

Online: Amazon.com; Whole Foods Market, local organic grocers/co-ops
Unbleached parchment paper muffin liners

REAL SALT

Online: realsalt.com, Amazon.com; grocery stores nationwide
Various unrefined salts

TROPICAL TRADITIONS

See also: Fats & Oils and Nuts
Online: tropicaltraditions.com
Cocoa powder, shredded coconut

WILDERNESS FAMILY NATURALS

Online: wildernessfamilynaturals.com
Organic raw cocoa powder, organic herbs & spices, natural unrefined salts

PANTRY ITEMS

BEAR & WOLF CANNED

Online: Amazon.com; Costco
Wild-caught salmon

BIONATURAE, JOVIAL, & POMI BRANDS

Online: tropicaltraditions.com; Whole Foods Market, local organic grocers/co-ops
Tomato products, strained tomatoes, chopped tomatoes

EMERALD COVE & EDEN FOODS

Grocery stores, Asian markets
Nori (dried seaweed paper)

IMPROVE'EAT

Online: improveat.com
Wraps

MEDITERRANEAN ORGANIC

Online: Amazon; local grocers
Olives, other grocery items—read labels

MOUNTAIN ROSE HERBS

Online: mountainroseherbs.com
Herbs & spices

SEASNAX

Online: seasnax.com; grocery stores

WILD PLANET

Online: Amazon.com; grocery stores
Canned sardines, wild-caught salmon

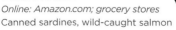

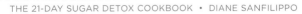

fats & oils

cleaning up your diet by using the right fats & oils is essential to improving your health

CHOOSING COOKING FATS

listed in order of most stable to least stable for cooking

The fats and oils are ranked below based on the following criteria: 1. how they're made—choose naturally occurring, minimally processed options first; 2. their fatty acid composition—the more saturated they are, the more stable and less likely to be damaged or oxidized they are; 3. their smoke point—which tells you how hot is too hot before the fats will be damaged, though smoke point should be considered a secondary factor to fatty acid profile.

WHICH TO EAT

SATURATED IDEAL FOR HOT USES
PLANT SOURCES *organic, unrefined forms are ideal*
coconut oil
palm oil *from sustainable sources*

ANIMAL SOURCES *pasture-raised/grass-fed & organic sources are ideal*

butter, ghee/clarified butter   schmaltz (chicken fat)
duck fat   tallow
lamb fat
lard

UNSATURATED IDEAL FOR COLD USES
organic, extra-virgin, & cold-pressed forms are ideal

avocado oil   nuts & seeds (including nut &
nut oils (walnut, pecan,   seed butters)
  macadamia)   flaxseed oil (higher in polyunsatu-
olive oil   rated fatty acids, so consume in
sesame oil   extremely limited amounts)

Note: Unsaturated fats—often called oils as listed above—are typically liquid at room temperature and are easily damaged (oxidized) when heat is applied to them. You do not want to consume damaged fats; therefore, cooking in these fats is not recommended.

WHICH TO DITCH

SATURATED
Man-made fats are never healthy. Trans fats are particularly harmful.
"Buttery spreads," including oil blends like Earth Balance, Benecol, and
  I Can't Believe It's Not Butter
hydrogenated or partially hydrogenated oils
margarine

UNSATURATED
These oils are highly processed and oxidize easily via one or more of the following: light, air, or heat. Consuming oxidized oils is never healthy.
canola oil (rapeseed oil)   safflower oil
corn oil   soybean oil
grapeseed oil   sunflower oil
rice bran oil   vegetable oil

For more detailed information on the fatty acid profiles of fats & oils, check out my book *Practical Paleo.*

VERY STABLE—IDEAL FOR COOKING

coconut oil
butter/ghee
cocoa butter
tallow/suet (beef fat)
palm oil *from sustainable sources*
lard/bacon fat (pork fat)
duck fat

MODERATELY STABLE—BEST COLD

avocado oil*
macadamia nut oil*
olive oil*
rice bran oil*

LEAST STABLE—NOT RECOMMENDED

safflower oil**
sesame seed oil*
canola oil**
sunflower oil**
vegetable shortening**
corn oil**
soybean oil**
walnut oil*
grapeseed oil**

*While not recommended for cooking, cold-pressed nut and seed oils that are stored in the refrigerator may be used to finish recipes or after cooking is completed, for flavor.

**These oils are not recommended for consumption, whether hot or cold, but are listed here for your reference, as they are commonly used.

quick-fix **meal math**

looking to make meals in minutes? check out this handy guide
to adding up protein, veggies, fat, and flavor to equal a quick bite!

PROTEIN + FAT + VEGGIE + FLAVOR = A QUICK-FIX MEAL!

Use any of your own favorites in this type of equation to create combinations that you enjoy.

 + **+** **+**

PROTEIN	FAT	VEGGIE	FLAVOR
- ground meat - hard-boiled eggs (HBE) - hot dogs* (grass-fed) - jerky* - turkey* - roast beef* (grass-fed) - rotisserie chicken or leftover cooked chicken** - sardines* (wild) - scrambled/fried eggs - salmon or tuna* (wild)	- avocado (AVO) or guacamole (GUAC) - coconut oil - Healthy Homemade Mayonnaise (HHM)* - extra-virgin olive oil (EVOO) - nuts or seeds (almonds, walnuts, sunflower seeds, etc.) - pesto*	- bell pepper - carrots - celery - cucumbers - lettuce - nori seaweed paper - raw sauerkraut* (KRAUT) - tomatoes - veggies, leftover from another meal or pre-cooked	- lemon or lime juice - hot sauce* - Sweetener-Free Ketchup* - mustard* - olives - pickles* - salad dressing* - spices

meal math **equation examples**

ground meat + coconut oil + veggies + spices

ground meat + AVO/GUAC + lettuce + hot sauce

HBE + HHM + cucumbers + pickles

HBE + GUAC + carrots + hot sauce

HBE + pesto + lettuce + spices

hot dog + bell pepper (bun) + KRAUT + mustard

hot dog + AVO + bell pepper (bun) + mustard

turkey + AVO/GUAC + KRAUT + hot sauce

turkey + HHM + KRAUT + pickles

turkey + AVO + carrots + salad dressing

roast beef + HHM + carrots + pickles

roast beef + GUAC + cucumbers + KRAUT + spices

sardines + EVOO + lettuce + hot sauce + lemon

sardines + AVO + bell pepper + hot sauce

scrambled/fried eggs + KRAUT + hot sauce

scrambled/fried eggs + AVO + veggies + spices

wild salmon/tuna + HHM + lettuce + pickles

wild salmon/tuna + EVOO + tomatoes + olives

wild salmon/tuna + AVO + cucumbers + mustard

wild salmon/tuna + HHM + cucumbers + hot sauce

*See pages 226-227 for a list of recommended products & brands or refer to the recipes in this book.

** Always check ingredients and buy only those made without unwanted oils (like canola, soybean, or vegetable oil) or other questionable ingredients.

 www.pinterest.com/21daysugardetox
There are countless ideas for meals and snacks throughout our Pinterest boards—hop online and check them out!

starchy **carbohydrate vegetables**

additional carb sources for those who are following the Energy Modifications for all levels of The 21DSD program

ITEM NAME	CARBS PER 100G	FIBER PER 100G	CARBS PER 1 CUP	OTHER NOTABLE NUTRIENTS
cassava (raw)	38g	2g	78g	Vitamin C, Thiamin, Folate, Potassium, Manganese
taro root	35g	5g	46g, sliced	B6, Vitamin E, Potassium, Manganese
plantain	31g	2g	62g, mashed	Vitamin A (beta carotene), Vitamin C, B6, Magnesium, Potassium
yam	27g	4g	37g, cubed	Vitamin C, Vitamin B6, Manganese, Potassium
white potato	22g	1g	27g, peeled	trace Vitamin C
sweet potato	21g	3g	58g, mashed	Vitamin A (beta carotene), Vitamin C, B6, Potassium, Manganese, Magnesium, Iron, Vitamin E
parsnips	17g	4g	27g, sliced	Vitamin C, Manganese
lotus root	16g	3g	19g, sliced	Vitamin C, B6, Potassium, Copper, Manganese
winter squash	15g	4g	30g, cubed	Vitamin C, Thiamin, B6
onion	10g	1g	21g, chopped	Vitamin C, Potassium
beets	10g	2g	17g, sliced	Folate, Manganese
butternut squash	10g	-	22g	Vitamin A (beta carotene), Vitamin C

recipe **index**

MAIN **DISHES**

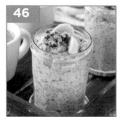
banana vanilla bean n'oatmeal

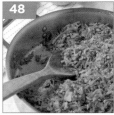
carrot-apple skillet breakfast hash

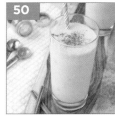
apple ginger green smoothie

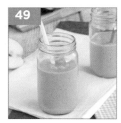
apple pie smoothie

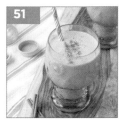
pumpkin spice smoothie

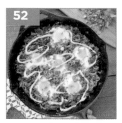
southwestern breakfast skillet

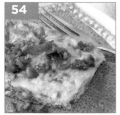
worth-the-wait crustless quiche

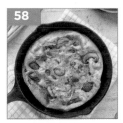
pizza frittata

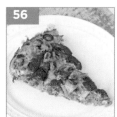
mushroom & green onion frittata

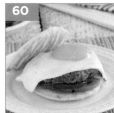
breakfast sausage & biscuit sandwich

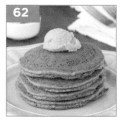
butternut squash pancakes

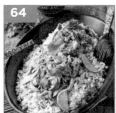
pollo asado

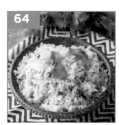
basic cilantro cauli-rice

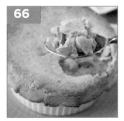
chicken pot pie

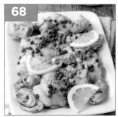
artichoke & lemon chicken with capers

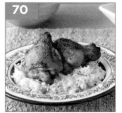
slow cooker chicken adobo

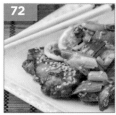
lemon ginger chicken

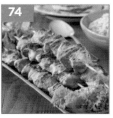
tandoori chicken skewers

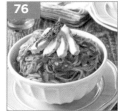
zoodles with creamy tomato sauce & chicken

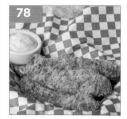
chicken strips

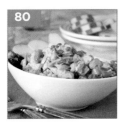
80
curried chicken salad
with apples

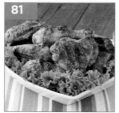
81
bbq chicken

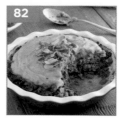
82
beef & bacon
cottage pie

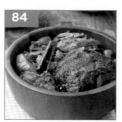
84
cinnamon & fennel
braised pork

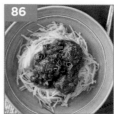
86
fennel & sage
meatballs

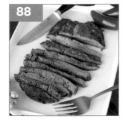
88
asian ginger flank
steak

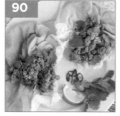
90
beef larb (thai
lettuce wraps)

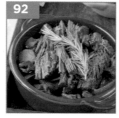
92
pot roast with
root veggies &
mushrooms

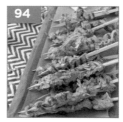
94
satay skewers

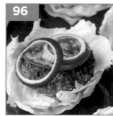
96
10-minute sliders

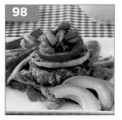
98
chorizo burgers with
spicy red onions

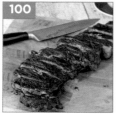
100
coffee & cocoa
rubbed ribs

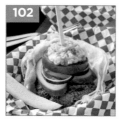
102
lamb burgers with
chunky avo-ziki

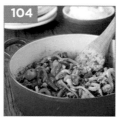
104
italian sausage &
peppers

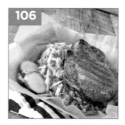
106
smoky grilled pork
chops with cookout
coleslaw

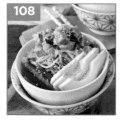
108
ahi tuna poke bowl

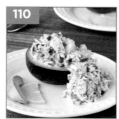
110
jalapeño-dill tuna
salad

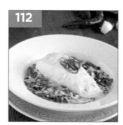
112
coconut-basil halibut
with spinach

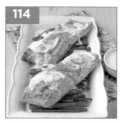
114
salmon with creamy
tzatziki sauce & dill
carrots

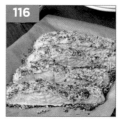
116
no-honey mustard
pecan-crusted
salmon

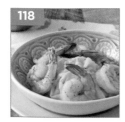
118
shrimp scampi
with creamy garlic
fettucine

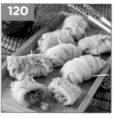
120
cabbage-wrapped
dumplings

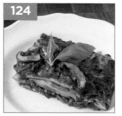
122
cilantro shrimp stir-
fry

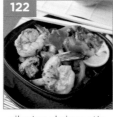
124
vegetable lasagne

SOUPS SALADS & **SIDES**

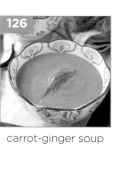

126
carrot-ginger soup

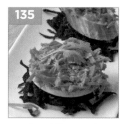

128
roasted cauliflower-leek soup

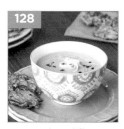

129
weeknight chicken soup

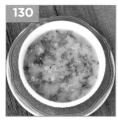

130
portuguese green soup (caldo verde)

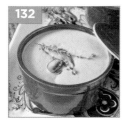

132
creamy mushroom soup

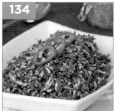

134
spicy slaw

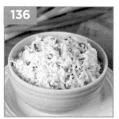

135
beet & carrot stacked salad

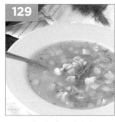

136
garlic & green onion cauli-rice

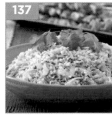

137
moroccan cauli-rice pilaf

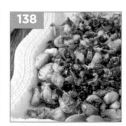

138
brussels sprouts with crispy capers & bacon

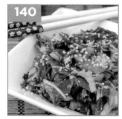

140
asian sautéed greens

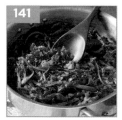

141
braised balsamic red cabbage

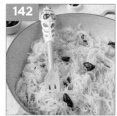

142
olive oil & garlic spaghetti

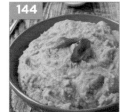

144
roasted butternut squash mash

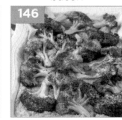

146
broccoli double take

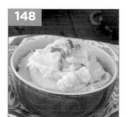

148
roasted garlic parsnip mash

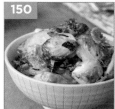

150
caramelized brussels sprouts & onions

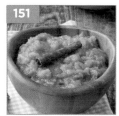

151
spiced applesauce

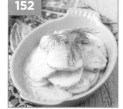

152
creamy cucumber salad

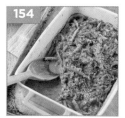

154
green bean casserole

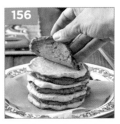
156

mini sweet potato
flatbreads

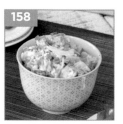
158

fennel & bacon
sweet potato salad

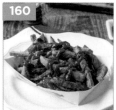
160

seasoned sweet
potato fries

SNACKS

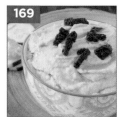
162

pesto deviled eggs

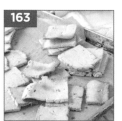
163

dill crackers

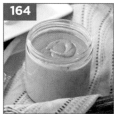
164

sunbutter

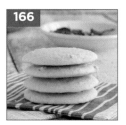
166

"buttermilk" buns

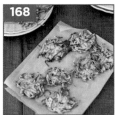
168

celery root cakes

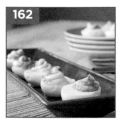
169

sundried tomato
hummus

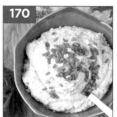
170

herb almond
"cheese" spread

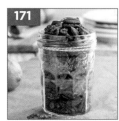
171

smoky lime nut mix

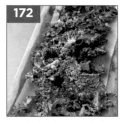
172

salt & vinegar kale
chips

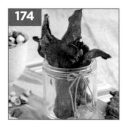
174

turkey jerky

NOT-SWEET **TREATS**

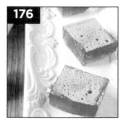
kombucha gelatin
176

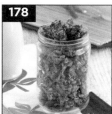
apple spice "granola"
178

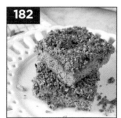
apple chai spice scones
180

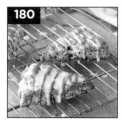
nutty cinnamon crumb cake
182

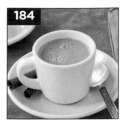
pumpkin spice latte
184

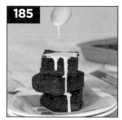
sunbutter brownies
185

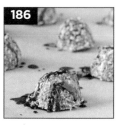
banana pecan macaroons with chocolate glaze
186

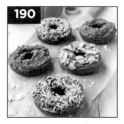
banana-nut cake mini donuts
188

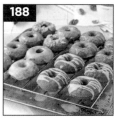
pumpkin spice donuts
190

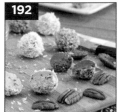
sunbutter truffles (cocoa-espresso & almond-cocoa nib)
192

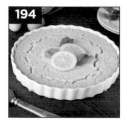
tart lemon torte
194

SAUCES & SPREADS

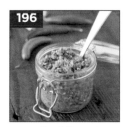
garlic chili paste
196

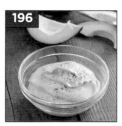
avocado crema
196

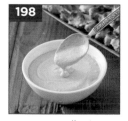
creamy cilantro garlic sauce
198

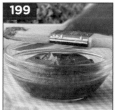
bbq sauce
199

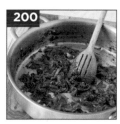
caramelized onions
200

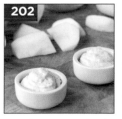
no-honey mustard sauce
202

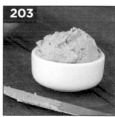
spiced buttery apple spread
203

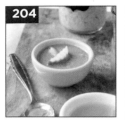
204

thousand island
dressing

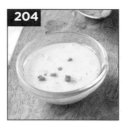
204

apple cider
vinaigrette

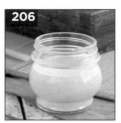
204

creamy ranch
dressing

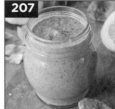
206

creamy pesto
dressing

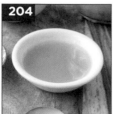
207

spinach & walnut
pesto

KITCHEN **BASICS**

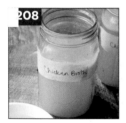
208

bone broth

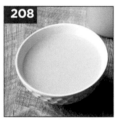
208

vegetable broth

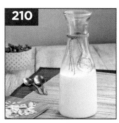
210

coconut milk

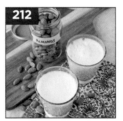
212

almond milk & meal

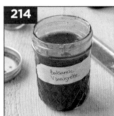
214

balsamic vinaigrette
dressing

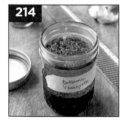
214

lemon-herb dressing

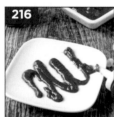
216

sweetener-free
ketchup

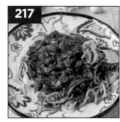
217

simple marinara

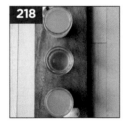
218

clarified butter &
ghee

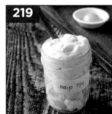
219

healthy homemade
mayonnaise

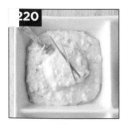
220

avo-goddess sauce

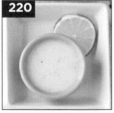
220

creamy ginger lime
dressing

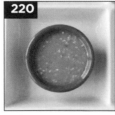
220

spicy sesame ginger
dressing

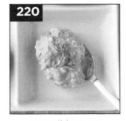
220

avo-ziki sauce

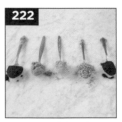
222

spice blends

ingredient index

nutrition facts for all recipes can be found online at balancedbites.com/21DSD

my thanks

"As we express our gratitude, we must never forget that the highest appreciation is not to utter words, but to live by them."
—John F. Kennedy

For those of you who are not aware, I brought Tonja Field onto my team to help work on this book—in tandem with me—so that I was able to complete it and deliver it to you in the time I planned on from the start. Writing, developing, cooking, and photographing recipes as just one person, working alone, well, that's no easy feat. And after completing all of that work solo for the first book, I decided that it was in the best interest of my own health and well-being—as well as the creativity and inspiration for recipes in this book—to invite someone along for the ride and to help me out.

Tonja

There aren't many words that I can use to express my gratitude to you beyond, quite simply, **thank you.**

When we started working on this project together, I knew that you were capable of helping to make it a more robust and creatively inspired resource than I could have created on my own. After finishing The 21DSD guidebook, I was worried I wouldn't be able to even conceptualize enough new recipes for this program to make this book come together. Despite the long hours, tiresome recipe testing, and stressful photo shoots, you completely came through with dedication and vigor I typically demand or expect only of myself. You treated this project as your own, and I'm truly grateful for that.

Together, we've produced a collection of recipes that will enhance the experience of 21DSDers around the world and bring tasty, sweetener-free, Paleo-friendly recipes to those who seek inspiration. I'm proud of this book, I'm proud of you, and I'm honored to have your love for food woven throughout these pages with mine.